Immunoassays for Drugs Subject to Abuse

Editors:

S. J. Mulé
Assistant Commissioner
New York State Drug Abuse Control Commission

I. Sunshine
Chief Toxicologist
Cuyahoga (Ohio) County Coroner's Office

M. Braude
Acting Chief
Preclinical Drug Studies Section
Center for Studies of Narcotic and Drug Abuse
National Institute on Drug Abuse

R. E. Willette
Chemist
Preclinical Drug Studies Section
Center for Studies of Narcotic and Drug Abuse
National Institute on Drug Abuse

published by

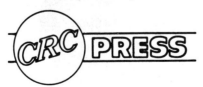

CRC PRESS, INC.
18901 Cranwood Parkway · Cleveland, Ohio 44128

©1974 by CRC Press, Inc.

International Standard Book Number 0-87819-121-6

Library of Congress Card Number 73-88630

Printed in the United States.

INTRODUCTION

The tremendous increase in the use and abuse of drugs by our society during the past decade has created a need for rapid, reliable, sensitive, specific and inexpensive methods to detect and identify drugs in biofluids. The major purpose of this analysis is to provide an objective measurement of drug and/or abuse. Such data would assist in the identification of the drug dependent person, evaluate objectively the progress of the patient in therapeutic treatment programs, and allow early detection and treatment of the drug abuser.

It is estimated at the present time that 15 to 20 million urine samples are being analyzed a year for drugs subject to abuse. Most of these tests are performed for chemotherapeutic treatment programs (e.g., methadone), the military, government, industry, law enforcement and correctional agencies. Obviously, urinalysis at this rate is quite costly and, therefore, must be used judiciously. Even so, the Federal government requires individuals within Methadone Maintenance Treatment Programs (MMTP) to be tested once each week for morphine and once each month for methadone, amphetamines and barbiturates.

The primary methods that have been used for the analysis of drugs subject to abuse are Thin-layer chromatography (TLC); Gas-liquid chromatography (GLC); and Spectrofluorometry (SPF). With the growing demand for rapid, convenient, and less expensive assay methods, considerable effort has been exerted in the past few years to improve on these existing methods and to develop new ones. This volume is directed towards the application of one of the new methods, the immunoassay, to the drug abuse field.

Immunoassay techniques were developed in 1960 to quantitatively measure insulin in human plasma. Since then, this technique has been applied successfully in clinical chemistry for the quantitative evaluation of a variety of compounds such as hormones, enzymes and drugs in biological fluids. With the increase in heroin and polydrug use as well as methadone maintenance treatment programs in the drug decade of the sixties, development of simple and sensitive techniques for the rapid evaluation of drugs of abuse in urine and biological fluids became necessary. However, it was not until the early 1970s that these immunoassay techniques were applied to the drug abuse field with the development of assays for morphine, barbiturates, methadone, mescaline pentazocine, amphetamine, LSD, etc.

In addition to the rapid development of immunoassays for a wide variety of drugs and other molecules of biological importance, there has been an important evolution of new immunochemical techniques. In the drug area, there are four different techniques currently available: the radioimmunoassay (RIA), the hemagglutination inhibition assay (HI), the enzyme multiplied immunoassay technique (EMIT), and the free radical assay technique (FRAT).

In general, the immunoassay techniques share the advantages of being relatively rapid and simple, adaptable to a large number of samples, and requiring a minimum of sample preparation. On the other hand, they vary considerably in sensitivity and are not as specific as other analytical methods, such as GLC and TLC. Positive results usually require a confirmatory test. At the present time, their costs are relatively high, but will lower with increases in volume of use.

It is still early to assess the full impact of immunoassays on the analysis of drugs, but it is already evident that it has provided an excellent method for handling large volumes of samples required for urinalysis screening programs.

During the period of preparation of this book, new immunoassays for drugs of abuse, such as marihuana and LSD, have become available, or are under development. Some of these immunoassays have recently been made available commercially in the form of kits. For instance, a hemagglutination assay kit for methadone has been marketed and one for benzoylecgonine (cocaine) is under development. A radioimmunoassay (RIA) kit for amphetamine and the first combination RIA kit, which will detect barbiturates and morphine (named mobarb), are in the final stages of field testing. In this rapidly developing area, new kits and techniques may be expected at an increasing rate. One can also expect an increase in the specificity of these assays, a reduction in cost, and the application of fully automated technology to this field in the near future.

Salvatore J. Mulé
Robert E. Willette

THE EDITORS

S. J. Mulé is Assistant Commissioner, New York State Drug Abuse Control Commission, Testing and Research Laboratory, Brooklyn. He received his B.A. degree from the College of Wooster, Ohio, his M.S. degree from Rutgers University, and his Ph.D. (Pharmacology) degree from the University of Michigan.

Irving Sunshine is Chief Toxicologist, Cuyahoga County Coroner's Office, Cleveland. He received his B.S., M.A., and Ph.D. degrees from New York University.

Monique C. Braude is Acting Chief, Preclinical Drug Studies Section, Center for Studies of Narcotic and Drug Abuse, National Institute on Drug Abuse, Rockville, Maryland. She received her M.S. degree from Ohio State University and her Ph.D. degree from the University of Maryland.

R. E. Willette is Chemist, Preclinical Drug Studies Section, Center for Studies of Narcotic and Drug Abuse, National Institute on Drug Abuse, Rockville, Maryland. He received his B.S. degree from Ferris State College and his Ph.D. (Pharmaceutical Chemistry) degree from the University of Minnesota.

CONTRIBUTORS

Dr. Frank L. Adler*
The Public Health Research
Institute of the City of New York
455 First Avenue
New York, New York 10016

Dr. Richard J. Bastiani
Syva Corporation
3181 Porter Drive
Palo Alto, California 94304

Dr. Milton L. Bastos
Toxicology Laboratory
Office Chief Examiner
520 First Avenue
New York, New York 10016

Dr. William Brattin
Cuyahoga County Coroner's Office
2121 Adelbert Road
Cleveland, Ohio 44106

Dr. Monique Braudé*
National Institute on Drug Abuse
5600 Fishers Lane
Rockville, Maryland 20852

Dr. Don H. Catlin*
Department of Pharmacology
UCLA School of Medicine
Los Angeles, California 90024

Dr. Michael H. Ebert*
Laboratory of Clinical Sciences
National Institute of Mental Health
Bethesda, Maryland 20014

Dr. Charles W. Gorodetzky*
Addiction Research Center
National Institute on Drug Abuse
P.O. Box 2000
Lexington, Kentucky 40507

Dr. Howard A. Gross*
Human Genetics Branch
National Institute of Dental Research
Bethesda, Maryland 20014

Dr. Stanley J. Gross*
Department of Pediatrics
UCLA School of Medicine
Los Angeles, California 90024

Dr. Richard L. Hawks*
Laboratory of Clinical Sciences
National Institute of Mental Health
Bethesda, Maryland 20014

Dr. Milton H. Joffe*
National Institute on Drug Abuse
5600 Fishers Lane
Rockville, Maryland 20852

Dr. Richard K. Leute
Syva Corporation
3181 Porter Drive
Palo Alto, California 94304

Dr. Lawrence Levine
Department of Biochemistry
Brandeis University
Waltham, Massachusetts 02154

Dr. Salvatore J. Mulé*
DACC Testing and Research Laboratory
80 Hanson Place
Brooklyn, New York 11217

Dr. Kenneth E. Rubenstein
Syva Corporation
3181 Porter Drive
Palo Alto, California 94304

Dr. Richard S. Schneider*
Syva Corporation
3181 Porter Drive
Palo Alto, California 94304

Mr. Arnold Seidner
Department of Physiological Chemistry
Roche Institute of Molecular Biology
Nutley, New Jersey 07110

Dr. James R. Soares
Department of Pediatrics
UCLA School of Medicine
Los Angeles, California 90024

Dr. Sydney Spector*
Department of Physiological Chemistry
Roche Institute of Molecular Biology
Nutley, New Jersey 07110

Dr. James L. Spratt*
Department of Pharmacology
University of Iowa
Iowa City, Iowa 52240

Dr. Irving Sunshine*
Cuyahoga County Coroner's Office
2121 Adelbert Road
Cleveland, Ohio 44106

Dr. Edwin F. Ullman
Syva Corporation
3181 Porter Drive
Palo Alto, California 94304

Dr. Helen VanVunakis*
Department of Biochemistry
Brandeis University
Waltham, Massachusetts 02154

Dr. Robert E. Willette*
National Institute on Drug Abuse
5600 Fishers Lane
Rockville, Maryland 20852

*Invited Conference Participants

This monograph consists of the proceedings of a one day meeting on Immunoassays for Drugs Subject to Abuse held under the sponsorship of the Center for Studies of Narcotic and Drug Abuse, National Institute of Mental Health (now, National Institute on Drug Abuse), Rockville, Maryland in March, 1973. The purpose of this meeting was to bring together a select group of outstanding clinical chemists, pharmacologists and others who are actively engaged in the development or the evaluation of immunoassay techniques for the detection of drugs of abuse. This Volume was assembled to bring workers in the field up to date on the application of novel analytical tools i.e., immunoassay techniques to the analysis of drugs of abuse. It was decided to limit the presentations to general methodologies and to essentially omit technical details as applied specifically to each drug of abuse, as these have already been published.

The structure of the meeting is clear from the Table of Contents of this volume, which closely follows the program outline. The 1-day meeting included 10 presentations: six of them focused on general principles of immunoassays and the various methodologies available, four of them were devoted to a critical evaluation of these methods and their specific application to the detection of drugs of abuse. Although attendance at the meeting was strictly limited to one scientist per laboratory, the papers in this volume represent usually the collaborative efforts of several scientists.

The subject matter in this monograph is arranged in a manner similar to the presentations at the conference, including: (1) A general introduction providing pertinent background information; (2) A review of the current state of the art of immunoassays from the theoretical as well as the practical standpoint; and (3) Critical evaluations of the various immunoassays for drugs of abuse as used in routine screening of biological materials with particular emphasis on comparisons with other established analytical techniques.

Presentations at the meeting were given by:

1. Dr. Frank L. Adler, Chief of the Department of Immunology, Public Health Research Institute of the City of New York, the developer of the hemagglutination inhibition (HI) technique.

2. Dr. Don H. Catlin, Assistant Professor in the Department of Pharmacology, UCLA School of Medicine, who has applied and critically evaluated immunoassay methods of the clinical level.

3. Dr. Charles W. Gorodetsky, Chief Section on Drug Metabolism and Kinetics, NIDA Addiction Research Center, Lexington, who has been involved in the clinical pharmacology and pharmacokinetics of drugs of abuse.

4. Dr. Stanley J. Gross, Research Pediatrician with the Department of Pediatrics, UCLA School of Medicine, who has been involved in the design of immunogens for steroids, marihuana and morphine.

5. Dr. Salvatore J. Mulé, Assistant Commissioner and Director of the New York State Drug Abuse Control Commission (DACC) Testing and Research Laboratory, one of the leading experts in the field of drug abuse analysis.

6. Dr. Richard S. Schneider, a Research Scientist at the Syva Company, who has been actively involved in the development of the Enzyme Multiplied Immunoassay Technique (EMIT) and the Free Radical Assay Technique (FRAT).

7. Dr. Sidney Spector, Senior Scientist, Roche Institute of Molecular Biology, who published the first immunoassay for morphine and has continued to contribute to this field.

8. Dr. James L. Spratt, Professor of Pharmacology at the University of Iowa, who is involved in the development of a solid-phase method for the immunoassay of morphine and other opiates.

9. Dr. Irving Sunshine, Chief Toxicologist, Cuyahoga County Coroner's Office and Professor of Toxicology at Case Western University, a leading expert in the area of bioanalytical and forensic methodology.

10. Dr. Helen Van Vunakis, Associate Professor, Brandeis University, Graduate Department of Biochemistry, whose interest in the mechanism of action of pharmacologically active compounds led her to produce specific antibodies

for narcotics, hallucinogens and neurotransmitters which are used in the development of immunological assays.

At the conference, Dr. Richard L. Hawks, a chemist and postgraduate fellow at the National Institute on Drug Abuse outlined the need for confirming the results, especially the positive findings, obtained by immunoassay methods, by using more specific analytical tools such as gas chromatography and mass spectrometry. Although this discussion did not fit per se in a book on immunoassay, it was considered of such practical importance by the editors that Dr. Hawks was invited to submit a paper on this subject.

Two of the original participants, Dr. Salvatore Mulé and Dr. Irving Sunshine served in a key role as editors of this book along with the two NIDA co-project officers, Dr. Monique C. Braude and Dr. Robert E. Willette.

A major contribution to this volume was the summaries of the discussions held after each paper, which were prepared by Drs. Mulé and Willette. Emphasis in the discussions was placed on the practical problems involved in the present methods, cost, quality control and future directions for research.

We hope that this interdisciplinary monograph will be helpful in bringing workers in the field up to date on these exciting new developments and that the information contained herein will be of value to pharmacologists, toxicologists, forensic scientists, clinical chemists and clinicians who have a primary concern or responsibility for the analysis of psychoactive drugs.

We acknowledge the contributions of many individuals, authors, discussants, administrators, consultants, and staff whose unselfish efforts made this book possible, and are grateful to the CRC Press for their assistance and excellent editorial support.

Monique C. Braude
Irving Sunshine

TABLE OF CONTENTS

IMMUNOASSAYS:
CURRENT STATE OF THE ART

HAPTEN DETERMINANTS AND PURITY – THE KEY TO IMMUNOLOGIC SPECIFICITY

S. J. Gross and J. R. Soares

TABLE OF CONTENTS

INTRODUCTION

Immunological approaches to detect and quantitate polypeptides,[1-5] steroids,[6-20] and more recently, drugs[21-31] are employed in research and clinical laboratories. The list of immune assays for other molecules is ever-growing.* The in vivo use of derivative haptens and antigens occurred earlier but has been less emphasized than their use for in vitro analysis.[32-39] Although the binding sites of IgG are becoming fairly well localized and assigned to its hypervariable region, controversy persists as to whether the usual diversity of the immune response is due to many different (somatic) genes functioning in an ordered manner or is caused by hypermutability of a few genes in the germ line. Current theories fitting either rationale fail as yet to reconcile the exquisite sensitivity and multiple specificities of the immune response observed in the laboratory. Since antibodies may be awesome

*The references cited are not intended to represent an exhaustive compilation.

in their ability to discriminate single atomic substitutions, indeed even discrete steric differences, let us briefly examine the factors found to be necessary to achieve specificity and review potential applications of immune models to the clinical situation using a variety of drugs.

REQUIREMENTS FOR A SPECIFIC IMMUNE RESPONSE

It has long been recognized that one can link a hapten to a macromolecule, inject the conjugate into an immunologically competent animal, and harvest antibodies which include those to the hapten moiety.[40] The subject animal must be genetically a "responder" with respect to the particular macromolecule carrier and to the hapten moiety of the immunogenic conjugate. At first glance it would seem most efficient to link the hapten by any of its available chemically reactive functions to the selected carrier molecule (e.g., protein, polypeptide, carbohydrate). Unfortunately, no matter how many competent animals are immunized with such an immunogenic conjugate, the antisera thus produced cannot contain a population in the total IgG pool which will recognize the chemically reactive group used for coupling to the carrier portion of the conjugate.[6,7] If only a few determinant groups exist in the native state then the loss of even one group can be critical.

The requirement that functional groups of the hapten remain unblocked in the conjugate was presaged by us in 1968 when we first reported on attempts to raise antibody to haptens having *selected* determinants known to be associated with physiological activity (estradiol C-17).[8] The crude results then obtained were refined in later work.[41]

Subsequent work with steroids and drugs made us (SJG) aware that not only those chemical functions primarily responsible for metabolic activity but *all* active functions of a small hapten must remain accessible in the hapten carrier conjugate to acquire the most exquisitely specific IgG populations of which the immune system is capable. Thus determinant groups relatively distant to fixed, insolubilized "receptor" recognition sites may be of major importance to immunological specificity expressed in response to a relatively rigid hapten containing only a small number of determinant functions and whose dimensions do not exceed the binding site of soluble IgG. The fewer the active functions available to serve as haptenic determinants, the more molecules of similar basic structure will be recognized by the antiserum. Blockade of a single hydroxyl group of morphine in the preparation of a morphine immunogen results in an antiserum which is entirely unable to distinguish homologous morphine from its surrogates with 0 to 2 absent or unavailable hydroxyl(s).[21] Antiserum produced by immunization with such a morphinyl immunogen reacts with codeine equally or better than with morphine. Similarly, heroin is not discriminated at all and dextromethorphan is not distinguished adequately. Blockade of a distant morphine hydroxyl function results in an IgG pool which apparently reacts to a significant degree with major variants at the tertiary nitrogen function. Indeed, even meperidine is recognized by this type of antiserum.

On cursory consideration such broad antibody recognition may seem to have merit. However, for precise assay work and for meaningful in vivo probes, much greater specificity is necessary. Increase in distance from the hapten moiety to the carrier by the simple device of lengthening the intermediate linking group on the reactive function may improve results but is not an adequate solution.[25] Certain ring linkages may have determinants chemically free but introduce new, perhaps significant ones.[16-20] All chemically reactive functions of a pure derivative, not only those which coincide with physiological activity, must remain undistorted and accessible to avail themselves as immunological determinants. There has been an increasing awareness and confirmation of this concept.

A pertinent recently published work concerned a serotonin conjugate[42] albeit omitting the rationale of synthesis and failing to take cognizance of the additional critical requirement of antigen purity. The hapten macromolecule conjugate should be highly pure to achieve an optimally specific immune response.

IgG purity (a selected IgG population) can be another factor useful in immunological assay procedures especially to assist in discriminating similar concentrations of homologous and heterologous haptens in a sample. Even if antiserum is generated by an ideally conceived and thoroughly purified antigen conjugate, it will contain inevitably an antibody population heterogeneous with respect to titer, K_a (average binding constant), and specificities. In the laboratory we generally accept this heterogeneity even if a high titer, high affinity antiserum is produced by a unique animal expressing a fortuitous genetic message. Naturally, such success is most likely if the immunogenic conjugate is correctly conceived, synthesized, and purified.

An eventual "good" animal response is virtually certain using routine immunization procedures. Specificity should persist and will do so (independent of titer[43]) over a prolonged immunization time course with a suitable immunogen.[44] This is an important factor for repeatable data. However, certain antigens are reported to deteriorate in this respect.[20] There are obvious possible explanations for the latter phenomenon which cannot be considered here.

CROSS-REACTIONS

Antibodies to a given hapten are heterogeneous in amino acid sequences and in affinities for the hapten. The K_a of the more specific IgG is greater than that of the less specific (or inert) IgG for a homologous hapten. If antibody is present in sufficient concentration, heterologous haptens will fail to cross-react completely even in marked hapten excess. This immunochemical criterion of antibody specificity is often overlooked. When an antiserum is completely inhibited by a heterologous hapten at a similar or even an order of

magnitude greater concentration than homologous hapten, the *relative* K_a's of available antibodies are not sufficiently dissimilar with respect to the two haptens and the conformation to determinants at the binding sites is relatively nonspecific. However, it should be emphasized that K_a is not synonymous with specificity. Its value can be high and the system reflect nonspecific binding or the value can be low and marked specificity be inherent. Since K_a of an antibody should be higher with respect to a homologous hapten than a heterologous one, K_a values are only meaningful when comparing the binding of antibody to two or more substrate haptens.

It has been shown that antibodies generated by a fairly rigid hapten with a limited number of available functional groups strikingly differ in binding to a heterologue having but one function less than the homologue.[44] A rationale for this experimental observation is provided by theoretical calculation indicating that the K_a for the hapten lacking a single critical hydroxyl group should be several hundredfold less than that for the homologue.

If the difference in the energy of these antibody hapten interactions (ΔF) relates to the energy of a single hydrogen bond and hydrogen bond energies range from 2 to 10 kcals per mol,[45] then the ratio of K homologue to K heterologue at 25°C may be calculated as follows using an intermediate energy value of 5 kilocals per mole:

$$\Delta F_{Homologue} - \Delta F_{Heterologue} = -(RT \ln K_{Homologue} - RT \ln K_{Heterologue})$$
$$\text{i.e., } -5{,}000 = -[1.987 \times 298 \times 2.3 \log (K_{Homologue}/K_{Heterologue})]$$
$$K_{Homologue}/K_{Heterologue} = 4.691 \times 10^3$$

Partial steric hindrance by an extra function is less relevant than absence of an important determinant. Thus a heterologous hapten containing an extra function would be expected to result in a less strikingly different K_a ratio than in the foregoing calculation. The precise nature of the functional group determinants, their accessibility, and solvent solubilities significantly bear on the ultimate K_a ratios.

ANTIBODY PURIFICATION

When crude antiserum of appropriate K_a, titer and specificity is achieved[43,46] we may select a

unique antibody population to avoid contributions by less useful IgG.[47] The crude serum sample is passed through a column or slurry of an insoluble matrix-hapten conjugate synthesized with the same constraints and care as was the immunogen.[31,48] Yields of active antibody average 90% of theoretical. Naturally such a select IgG population which discriminates isomers and single atomic substitutions does not exist in crude antisera if critical hapten functions were rendered inaccessible in preparation of the conjugate used as the immunogen. One or a thousand host animals immunized with such material would fail to produce the required antibody. Of course, an impure antigen also may contribute to failure.[49]

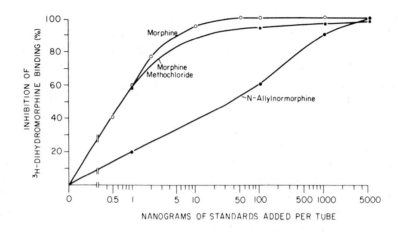

FIGURE 1. Inhibition of 7 to 8 ^{3}H dihydromorphine binding to azomorphine antiserum by morphine and related N-substituted alkaloids. Increased steric hindrance at the tertiary nitrogen (N-allylnormorphine) resulted in 100-fold average decrease in antiserum affinity for hapten. The quaternary nitrogen of morphine methochloride was recognized by only certain antibody populations.

IN VITRO, IMMUNE ASSAYS

Morphine

Antisera* raised by keyhole limpet hemocyanin (KLH), bovine serum albumin (BSA) or synthetic polypeptides coupled to morphine and heroin through the aromatic ring of the hapten by a small (e.g., para-aminobenzoic acid (PABA)) or large (PABA – polypeptide) diazonium ion results in antisera which not only detect morphine in the low picogram/ml range (sensitivity is primarily dependent on the ratio of hapten moieties per carrier molecule, immune schedule, and individual immune response), but more significantly, may discriminate between morphine, codeine, heroin, methadone, and dextromethorphan.[31] The latter two drugs can be present in 5- to 10,000-fold excess and remain unrecognized.[31] Further improvement can be expected by use of a homologous marker instead of the widely employed ^{3}H-dihydromorphine or ^{125}I-morphine, the former of which especially is sterically at variance with the native molecule. If the immunogenic conjugates are prepared in accordance with the foregoing constraints, even subtle alterations at the tertiary nitrogen can be detected (Figure 1).

Δ^9-Tetrahydrocannabinol (THC)

Antiserum** was raised employing an approach similar to the one described for morphine.[22,31] Specificities are shown in Figure 2. Figure 3 illustrates a standard curve by radioimmune assay used in the quantitation of THC in body fluids. Radioimmune specificities with respect to THC metabolites conform with the foregoing results and are to appear elsewhere.[44] An assay for general clinical purposes should be available shortly.*

Amphetamine and Phenobarbital

Clearly the foregoing principles are widely applicable and not restricted to any one metabolically significant substrate. Amphetamine and phenobarbital are simple additional examples. If the NH$_2$ function of amphetamine[30] is blocked, cross-reaction with methedrine is expected. If the aromatic moiety of phenobarbital is inaccessible[26] or its C-5 aliphatic sequence altered,[29] a less specific response to the relevant portion occurs. The foregoing principles applied to both these haptens result in conjugates which can generate

---

*Biological Developments, Inc.

**Biological Developments, Inc.

*Union Carbide Corp., Clinical Diagnostics Department.

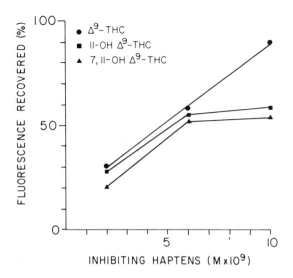

FIGURE 2. Inhibition of azoTHC quenching of antibody fluorescence by native Δ^9-THC and metabolites. Antibody IgG, purified by affinity chromatography, at 1 x 10^{-10} m/ml. (0.05 M sodium phosphate, pH 7.8) is maximally quenched (Qmax) by 5 x 10^{-10} m/ml azoTHC. Native cannabinoids, at various concentrations (abscissa), specifically inhibit azoTHC binding to antibody. Percent recovery of fluorescence = [(Qmax − Q_i)/Q_m] x 100%, where Q_i is the quenching observed in the presence of inhibitor. Antibody shows greatest recognition of Δ^9-THC, while lesser specificity is apparent for 11-hydroxy-THC and 8,11-dihydroxy-THC.

antisera** specific for the homologue and which can detect subtle differences in similar native haptens. It was not unexpected that phenobarbital antiserum distinguishes the phenyl substituent

(Figure 4). However, it is interesting that even crude antiserum from an initial bleeding detects slight differences in the C-5 side chains. Amphetamine antiserum failed appreciably to recognize methedrine (Figure 5). Note that the inhibition curves for dextro and levo amphetamine isomers are quite distinctive using the crude antiserum.

ALTERNATIVE IMMUNE ASSAYS

There have been other less sensitive but interesting immune techniques brought to bear on body fluid assays. These include spin resonance[28] and enzyme[50] methods described elsewhere in this text. "Receptor" (circulating and cellular supernate) assays[51-53] are reported to be highly sensitive but many workers have experienced difficulties in reducing this approach to routine clinical practice. Undoubtedly as more "receptors" are isolated, more will be heard about nonimmune ligand binding assays. Fluorescence perturbations including decay alterations are extremely sensitive and specific indicators of substrate binding to macromolecules. Our laboratory has compiled measurements of fluorescence quenching of antibody[22] and fluorescence enhancement of hapten.[41] If the binding is specific and rigorous spectroscopic criteria are met (the emission wavelength of antibody overlaps the absorbance (excitation) peak of hapten) one can quantitate specific fluorescence intensity changes.[54,56] *Inhibition* of antibody fluorescence,[41] *inhibition* of fluores-

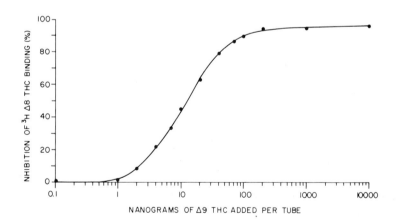

FIGURE 3. THC standard curve. Binding of ^{3}H-Δ^8-THC is inhibited with increasing amounts of unlabeled Δ^9-THC.

**Biological Developments, Inc.

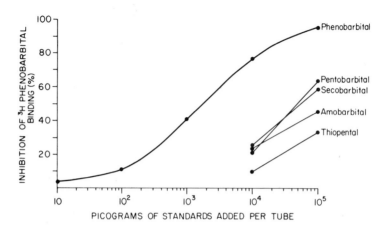

FIGURE 4. Radioimmunoassay demonstrates that crude phenobarbital antiserum clearly distinguishes phenobarbital from other barbiturates lacking the phenyl ring. Subtle differences are detected in the other barbiturates tested.

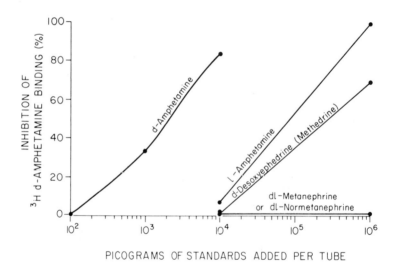

FIGURE 5. d-Amphetamine antiserum has minimal cross-reactivity (0.07%) with methedrine by radioimmunoassay. l-Amphetamine is recognized less than the d-homologue by crude antiserum. Its cross-reactivity is 4.5%.

cence enhancement[41] (or polarization[57,58]) of a fluorescent hapten, and finally, *interference* with the fluorescence decay by native haptens form the main basis of immune fluorescence *assays*. These techniques are simple, extremely rapid, and specific. Changes in fluorescence intensity and wavelength depend on rapid conformational changes occurring mainly at specific binding sites and not at nonspecific sites. Since a significant perturbation occurs only if the precise binding site of antibody is hit by a hapten absorbing or exciting at an optimal wavelength, the background binding to inert proteins or polypeptides is low. However, fluorescence by nonspecific proteins or other fluorescent spacing and binding of markers to anionic "receptors" in the sample is a major concern, especially if emission measurements are made toward the red (e.g., 420 nm or less). At present, considerable effort is being exerted to diminish this problem.

IN VIVO PROBES:
THC AND MORPHINE

Immunization against small steroid hormones historically has long been used in the laboratory to obtain in vivo metabolic data.[33-35] Recognizing that the results thus far have not been very fruitful, it is important not to overlook that active immunization with an immunogen or passive introduction of an antibody (cell) preparation as metabolic probes have the same rigorous constraints pertaining to specificity as in assay work. There is a compelling rationale for this view in providing meaningful metabolic results.[31,37,39]

While it is plausible to set up an arbitrary competition between circulating antibodies and fixed tissue "receptors," such an artificial in vivo experiment need not produce stoichiometric results. It has been assumed by some workers that antibodies could not theoretically be expected to compete successfully with (fixed) "receptors" because of unfavorable K_a values. However, there are major potential fallacies in mathematical calculations of such constants.[43] Indeed, even if the systems under consideration were homogenous and the binding site numbers known, comparing the affinities of fixed macromolecules to soluble (and heterogeneous) antibodies may be invalid.

In point of fact, the competition between fixed receptors and soluble antibodies may not transpire effectively since the hapten-antibody complex may be cleared. Certainly the hapten-antibody complex would be expected to retard hapten access in appreciable concentration, if at all, to fixed CNS receptors across the blood brain barrier. Methods may be designed to alter a finite pharmacological effect of a subsequently introduced homologous metabolic agent. It has been postulated that the circulating hapten-protein complex may serve either as an immunogen or a reservoir for active hapten.[38] Thus, it would seem that cross purposes could be served.

In the light of the foregoing perspective, we reported that a markedly ameliorated drug (THC) effect follows active immunization against the homologous hapten.[37] In this early, preliminary work, the thermoregulatory responses of rats to THC were almost entirely obliterated after one or two courses of active immunization with a THC-KLH conjugate. Subsequently, using a specific morphine immunogen we observed a marked general reduction of the analgesic effect of morphine. The analgesic blockade usually was accompanied by a remarkable syndrome at the time of challenge with native morphine, not seen in the THC experiments, and clinically best described as a hypersensitivity or withdrawal-like phenomenon.[39] These observations are at variance with the results of others.[36,38] The clinical observations were paralleled by antibody levels. Immune clearance (see review by Weigle[59]) and hypersensitivity experiments were not done in these limited studies undertaken for feasibility purposes. Passive transfer experiments and results of long-term active immunization have not yet been reported by us but the early data suggest that the foregoing immunologic techniques can be useful as metabolic probes in vivo, provided the proper immunogenic preparations are selected.

CONCLUSION

A hapten-directed antibody response requires the subject to respond to both the carrier and the hapten moieties of an immunogenic conjugate. Specificity of the hapten-directed antibody is dictated primarily by the restricted number and characteristics of available haptenic determinants. When an antiserum is directed to a hapten, one or more of whose determinant groups were inaccessible on the immunogen, immune assay data clearly demonstrate IgG populations of broad, low specificity. In such systems, homologous and heterologous haptens of similar basic structures rapidly and in relatively low concentrations compete on a more or less equal basis.

Since cross-reacting metabolites and experimental errors may provide additive errors, future diagnostic in vitro and metabolic in vivo studies will require highly specific reagents.

To achieve the most meaningful results, a well-conceived and pure immunogenic conjugate containing sufficient and appropriate hapten determinants provides the major key to a hapten-specific immune response.

REFERENCES

1. **Berson, S. A. and Yalow, R. S.,** Quantitative aspects of the reaction between insulin and insulin-binding antibody, *J. Clin. Invest.,* 38, 1996, 1959.

2. **Odell, W. D., Ross, G. R., and Rayford, P. L.,** Radioimmunoassay for luteinizing hormone in human plasma or serum: Physiological studies, *J. Clin. Invest.,* 46, 248, 1967.

3. **Unger, R. H., Eisentraut, A. M., McCall, M. S., and Madison, L. L.,** Glucagon antibodies and an immunoassay for glucagon, *J. Clin. Invest.,* 40, 1180, 1961.

4. **Heding, L.,** Radioimmunological determination of pancreatic and gut glucagon in plasma, *Diabetologia,* 7, 10, 1971.

5. **Rose, J. C. and Newsome, H. H., Jr.,** The rapid production of antisera to ACTH, angiotensin II and deoxycorticosterone with sufficient sensitivity for use in radioimmunoassays, *J. Clin. Endocrinol. Metab.,* 35, 469, 1972.

6. **Goodfriend, L. and Sehon, A. H.,** Preparation of an estrone-protein conjugate, *Can. J. Biochem. Physiol.,* 36, 1177, 1958.

7. **Beiser, S. M., Erlanger, B. F., Agate, F. J., and Lieberman, S.,** Antigenicity of steroid-protein conjugates, *Science,* 129, 564, 1959.

8. **Gross, S. J., Campbell, D. H., and Weetall, H. H.,** Production of antisera to steroids coupled to proteins directly through the phenolic A ring, *Immunochemistry,* 5, 55, 1968.

9. **Oliver, G. C., Jr., Parker, B. M., Brasfield, D. L., and Parker, C. W.,** The measurement of digitoxin in human serum by radioimmunoassay, *J. Clin. Invest.,* 47, 1035, 1968.

10. **Midgley, A. R., Jr., Niswender, G. D., and Ram, J. S.,** Hapten radioimmunoassay: A general procedure for the estimation of standard and other haptenic substances, *Steroids,* 13, 731, 1969.

11. **Midgley, A. R., Jr. and Niswender, G. D.,** Radioimmunoassay of Steroids. Karolinska Symposia on Research Methods in Reproductive Endrocrinology, 2nd Symposium Steroid Assay by Protein Binding, March 23, 1970.

12. **Africa, R. and Haber, E.,** The production and characterization of specific antibodies to aldosterone, *Immunochemistry,* 8, 479, 1970.

13. **Smith, T. W., Butler, V. P., Jr., and Haber, E.,** Characterization of antibodies of high affinity and specificity for the digitalis glycoside digoxin, *Biochemistry,* 9, 331, 1970.

14. **Ito, T., Woo, J., Haning, R., and Horton, R.,** A radioimmunoassay for aldosterone in human peripheral plasma including a comparison of alternate techniques, *J. Clin. Endocrinol.,* 34, 106, 1972.

15. **Gross, S. J., Grant, J. D., Bennett, R., Wong, R., and Lomax, P.,** Estriol-specific antibody for steroid assays, *Steroids,* 18, 555, 1971.

16. **Exley, D., Johnson, M. W., and Dean, P. D. G.,** Antisera highly specific for 17β estradiol, *Steroids,* 18, 605, 1971.

17. **Jeffcoate, S. L. and Searle, J. E.,** Preparation of a specific antiserum to estradiol-17β coupled to protein through the B ring, *Steroids,* 19, 181, 1971.

18. **Lindner, H. R., Perl, E., Friedlander, A., and Zeitlin, A.,** Specificity of antibodies to ovarian hormones in relation to the site of attachment of the steroids to the peptide carrier, *Steroids,* 19, 357, 1971.

19. **Kuss, E. and Goebel, R.,** Determination of estrogens by radioimmunoassay with antibodies to estrogen C6-conjugates. I. Synthesis of estrone, estradiol-17β and estriol-6-albumin conjugates, *Steroids,* 19, 509, 1972.

20. **Walker, C. S., Clark, S. J., and Wotiz, H. H.,** Factors involved in the production of specific antibodies to estriol and etradiol, *Steroids,* 21, 259, 1972.

21. **Spector, S. and Parker, C. W.,** Morphine: Radioimmunoassay, *Science,* 168, 1347, 1970.

22. **Grant, J. D., Gross, S. J., Lomax, P., and Wong, R.,** Antibody detection of marihuana, *Nat. New Biol.,* 236, 216, 1972.

23. **Spector, S.,** Quantitative determination of morphine in serum by radioimmunoassay, *J. Pharmacol. Exp. Ther.,* 178, 253, 1971.

24. **van Vunakis, H., Wasserman, E., and Levine, L.,** Specificities of antibodies to morphine, *J. Pharmacol. Exp. Ther.,* 180, 514, 1972.

25. **Wainer, B. H., Fitch, F. W., Rothberg, R. M., and Fried, J.,** Morphine-3-succinyl bovine serum albumin. An immunogenic hapten protein conjugate, *Science,* 176, 1143, 1972.

26. **Flynn, E. J. and Spector, S.,** Determination of barbiturate derivatives by radioimmunoassay, *J. Pharmacol. Exp. Ther.,* 181, 547, 1972.

27. **Peskar, B. A., Peskar, B. M., and Levine, L.,** Specificities of antibodies to normetanephrine, *Eur. J. Biochem.,* 26, 191, 1972.

28. **Leute, R. K., Ullman, E. F., Goldstein, A., and Herzenberg, L. A.,** Spin immunoassay technique for determination of morphine, *Nature,* 93, 236, 1972.

29. **Chung, A., Kim, S. Y., Cheng, L. T., and Castro, A.,** Phenobarbital specific antisera and radioimmunoassay, *Nature,* in press.

30. **Voss, E. W. and Berger, B. B.,** Neutralization of LSD by active immunization, personal communication.

31. **Gross, S. J., Grant, J. D., Wong, R., Schuster, R., Lomax, P., Campbell, D. H., and Bennett, R.,** Critical determinants enabling an antibody to distinguish morphine from heroin, codeine and dextromethorphan, *Immunochemistry,* in press

32. Landsteiner, K., Experiments on anaphylaxis to azoproteins, *J. Exp. Med.,* 39, 631, 1924.

33. Neri, R. O., Tolksdorf, S., Beiser, S. M., Erlanger, B. F., Agate, F. J., Jr., and Lieberman, S., Further studies on the biological effects of passive immunization with antibodies to steroid-protein conjugates, *Endocrinology,* 74, 593, 1964.

34. Perin, M., Zimmering, P. E., and Vande Wiele, R. L., Effects of antibodies to 17β-estradiol on PMS-induced ovulation in immature rats, *Endocrinology,* 94, 893, 1960.

35. Curd, J., Smith, T. W., Jaton, J-C., and Haber, E., The isolation of digoxin-specific antibody and its use in reversing the effects of digoxin, *Proc. Natl. Acad. Sci. U.S.A.,* 68, 2401, 1971.

36. Berkowitz, B. A. and Spector, S., Antibodies to morphine: Production of partial immunity to narcotics, *Abstr. V. Int. Cong. Pharmacol.,* 19, 1972.

37. Lomax, P., Gross, S. J., and Campbell, C., Immunological blockade of the hypothermic effects of Δ⁹-tetrahydrocannabinol in the rat, in, *The Pharmacology of Thermoregulation,* Schönbaum, E. and Lomas, P., Eds., Karger, Basel, 1973, 488.

38. Berkowitz, B. A. and Spector, S., Evidence for active immunity to morphine in mice, *Science,* 178, 1290, 1972.

39. Lomax, P., Campbell, C., and Gross, S. J., Immunological blockade of the analgesic effect of morphine in the rat, *Proc. West. Pharmacol. Soc.,* 16, 252, 1972.

40. Landsteiner, K. and van der Scheer, J., On crossreaction of immune sera to azoproteins, *J. Exp. Med.,* 63, 325, 1936.

41. Gross, S., Specificities of steroid antibodies, in, *Immunologic Methods in Steroid Determination,* Peron, F. G. and Caldwell, B. V., Eds., Appleton-Century Crofts, New York, 1970, 41.

42. Peskar, B. and Spector, S., Serotonin: Radioimmunoassay, *Science,* 174, 1340, 1973.

43. Grant, J. D. and Gross, S. J., Critical attributes of antisera for immunoassay, in preparation.

44. Wong, S. R., Soares, J. R., Gross, S. J., and Grant, J. D., Assay of plasma estriol by azoestriol antiserum without chromatography, in preparation.

45. Pauling, L., *The Nature of the Chemical Bond,* 3rd. ed., Cornell University Press, Ithaca, New York, 1960, 469.

46. Coligan, J. E., Egan, M. L., and Todd, C. W., Detection of carcinoembryonic antigen by radioimmune assay, *Natl. Cancer Inst. Monogr.,* 35, 427, 1972.

47. Gross, S. J. and Grant, J. D., In vitro recognition of diethylstilbestrol by anti-azobenzoyl estradiol IgG, *Steroids,* 16, 387, 1970.

48. Weliky, N., Weetall, H. H., Gilden, R. V., and Campbell, D. H., *Immunochemistry,* 1, 214, 1964.

49. Campbell, D. H., On the significance of inhibiting haptens, *Ann. N.Y. Acad. Sci.,* 169, 105, 1970.

50. Rubenstein, K. E., Schneider, R. S., and Dilman, E. F., "Homogeneous" enzyme immunoassay, *Biochem. Biophys. Res. Commun.,* 47, 846, 1972.

51. Murphy, B. E. P., The determination of thyroxin by competitive protein-binding analysis employing an amine exchange resin and radiothyroxine, *J. Lab. Clin. Med.,* 66, 161, 1965.

52. Tulchinsky, D. and Korenmen, S. G., A radio-ligand assay for plasma estrone: Normal values and variations during the menstrual cycle, *J. Clin. Endocrinol.,* 31, 76, 1970.

53. Leftkowitz, R. J., Roth, J., and Pastan, I., Radioreceptor assay of adrenocorticotropic hormone: New approach to assay of polypeptide hormones in plasma, *Science,* 170, 633, 1970.

54. Stryer, L., The interaction of a naphthalene dye with apomyoglobin and apohaemoglobin. A fluorescence probe of non-polar binding sites, *J. Mol. Biol.,* 13, 482, 1965.

55. Velick, S. F., Parker, C. W., and Eisen, H. H., Excitation energy transfer and the quantitative study of the antibody hapten reaction, *Proc. Natl. Acad. Sci. U.S.A.,* 46, 1470, 1960.

56. Haber, E. and Richards, F. F., The specificity of antigenic recognition of antibody heavy chain, *Proc. R. Soc. Lond. B. Biol. Sci.,* 166, 176, 1966.

57. Portman, A. J., Levison, S. A., and Dandliker, W. B., Anti-fluorescein antibody of high affinity and restricted heterogeneity as characterized by fluorescence polarization and quenching equilibrium techniques, *Biochem. Biophys. Res. Commun.,* 43, 207, 1971.

58. Dandliker, W. B., Kelly, R. J., Dandliker, J., Farquhar, L., and Levin, L., Fluorescence polarization immunoassay. Theory and experimental method, *Immunochemistry,* 10, 219, 1973.

59. Weigle, W. D., Fate and biological action of antigen-antibody complexes, *Adv. Immunol.,* 1, 283, 1961.

RADIOIMMUNOASSAYS FOR MORPHINE

S. Spector and A. Seidner

TABLE OF CONTENTS

INTRODUCTION

One of the more exciting advances in the field of drug analysis has been the development of the radioimmunoassay technique. Originally described in 1960 by Yalow and Berson,[1] this technique has made available to the endocrinologist, physiologist, biochemist, and pharmacologist a very sensitive and specific method for the quantitative measurement of hormones, enzymes, and drugs in biological fluids.

The basic principle of radioimmunoassay utilizes the reaction between an antigen (or hapten) and an antibody. Small molecules such as drugs can serve as haptens and can usually be made antigenic by chemically coupling them to a macromolecular substance. Animals will develop antibodies to the injected immunogen as part of their natural immune response. The serum derived from these animals is used as the antibody source, and tested with reference to their specificity, affinity, and titer.

The reaction between the hapten molecule (both radioactive labeled and unlabeled) and antibody is shown in Figure 1. The hapten in the antibody complex is referred to as BOUND hapten, while the uncomplexed hapten is referred to as FREE hapten.

To perform a radioimmunoassay, a fixed quantity of antiserum containing the antibody is mixed with a constant amount of radioactive hapten and the sample containing the hapten to be measured. The antibody will react with both the radioactive and unlabeled hapten forming a hapten antibody complex. Since both radioactive and free hapten will compete for the limited number of antibody sites available, the amount of radioactivity that ultimately combines with the antibody will be an inverse factor of the amount of unlabeled hapten competing for this site. This is presented graphically in Figure 2.

In order to measure the radioactivity in the hapten antibody complex or the free hapten, a convenient means of separating these fractions is necessary. There are several methods of separation that are commonly used, such as precipitating the complex with ammonium sulfate, ethanol, another antibody (double antibody technique), or absorbing it on dextran-coated charcoal or on special filters. Following separation, either the hapten antibody complex or the free hapten fraction is counted and the counts are used to determine the hapten concentration. The basic steps for performing a typical radioimmunoassay are outlined in Figure 3 and described below.

In 1970, the first description of experimental production of antibodies with a specificity for morphine appeared as part of the development of a radioimmunoassay for morphine by Spector and Parker.[2] Subsequently, other morphine-protein derivatives were prepared by coupling bovine serum albumin to various sites on the morphine moiety. The preparation of these antigens and the specificities of the antibodies generated by them were discussed recently.[3] More detailed discussions on antibody specificity and the design of antigens will be found elsewhere in this text.

This approach was later extended to the barbiturates.[3,4] In this case, the barbiturate hapten moiety was conjugated to the protein through an alkyl side chain in the 5-position. The antibodies generated to this antigen could distinguish commonly abused barbiturates and other classes of structurally related sedatives and anticonvulsants.

Catlin et al.[5] described a modification of the assay originally described by Spector and Parker[2] for the analysis of morphine in urine and serum specimens.

The procedure outlined below is similar to that described by Catlin et al.[5] but utilizes a ^{125}I-labeled morphine rather than the tritium-labeled dihydromorphine.

METHODS

This procedure described is for untreated urine specimens. These specimens require no special handling. Pipetted samples should be free of gross debris.

Protocol

1. Tubes are set up and labeled for the morphine-positive control and for assays of unknown urine specimens. Because of the importance of control values in the determination, it is recommended that the positive control be done in triplicate.

2. 0.1 ml of morphine-positive urine control is added to each of three tubes.

3. 0.1 ml of each unknown urine specimen is added to remaining numbered tubes.

4. 0.2 ml morphine antibody reagent is added to each tube and the contents are mixed well on a Vortex mixer.

5. 0.2 ml ^{125}I-morphine reagent is added to each tube, and the contents are mixed well on a Vortex mixer. (The ^{125}I-morphine and the morphine antibody reagent may be premixed prior to performing the assay, thereby eliminating one pipetting step. For those who wish to premix these reagents, it is recommended that the reagents be premixed in equal volumes and kept at room

ANTIGEN ANTIBODY REACTION

Antibody (Ab)

+ +

Unlabeled Antigen (Ag)   Labeled Antigen (Ag*)

Ag Ab Complex   Ag*Ab Complex

FIGURE 1.

PRINCIPLE OF RADIOIMMUNOASSAY

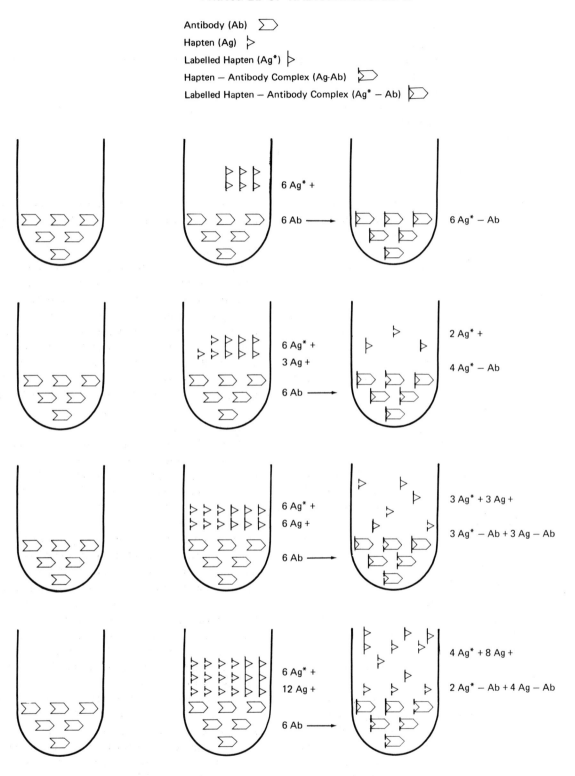

FIGURE 2.

BASIC PROCEDURE

1. Make up necessary reagents
2. Collect sample
3. Antibody (Ab) + Radioactive Antigen (Ag*) + sample (or standard)
4. Incubate
5. Separate Ag*Ab (bound) from Ag* (free)
6. Count radioactivity
7. Calculate results

FIGURE 3.

temperature for at least 1 day prior to their use. The incubation time, step 6, should be increased from at least 10 min to at least 1 hr in order to assure reproducible results.)

6. Tubes are incubated at ambient temperatures for 10 min.

7. 0.5 ml of the supernatant from a saturated ammonium sulfate solution is added to each tube to precipitate globulins. Each tubes's contents are then mixed well on a Vortex mixer.

8. Tubes are allowed to stand at ambient temperature for a minimum of ten minutes to complete precipitation.

9. Centrifuge for 10 min, at approximately 1,200 to 2,500 x g.

10. 0.5 ml of supernatant fluid is withdrawn from each tube without disturbing any precipitate along the sides or at the bottom of the tube (the supernatant fluid must be clear). It is transferred to a suitable vial for counting.

11. Each vial is counted in a gamma scintillation spectrometer for 1 min to obtain counts/min (CPM).

For higher cutoff levels — Should it be desirable to establish a cutoff level higher than 40 ng/ml, this can be done by diluting the urine sample with normal human urine and using 0.1 ml of the diluted sample in Step 3 of the Test Procedure (e.g., a dilution of 1:5 will provide a cutoff level of 200 ng/ml).

Alternatively, the use of smaller volumes of the sample urine instead of dilution of urine may be used to achieve a higher cutoff level. Positive urine controls containing higher concentrations of morphine should be used when this is done, i.e., a 100-ng/ml control or a 200-ng/ml control may be substituted for the 40-ng/ml control. To use the 100-ng/ml cutoff, 0.04 ml must be substituted for

the 0.1-ml volume of the sample and control. A 0.02-ml volume is used for the 200-ng/ml cutoff.

Evaluation

Counts per minute obtained from each unknown specimen are compared with average CPM obtained from morphine—positive controls.

Negative results — The test is negative for the presence of morphine when the CPM of the unknown specimen are lower than that of the average CPM of the morphine-positive control.

Positive results — The test is positive when the unknown specimen CPM are equal to or higher than that of the average CPM of the morphine-positive control.

The radioimmunoassay (RIA) for morphine protocol presented above describes a qualitative test. If there is need of quantitation, the following modification of the above procedure may be used to establish a standard curve in place of only positive controls.

Quantitative test — The ability to quantitate radioimmunoassay results is facilitated by running a standard curve in the range of the concentration being measured (Figure 4). This is simply done by substituting standard solutions of the material being measured in known concentrations and measuring the radioactivity at these concentrations. A standard curve is plotted using a value related to radioactivity as one axis and concentration as the second axis.

To establish a standard curve — The normal urine control is used as the O point on the standard curve and as the diluent for preparing standard solutions. A known amount of morphine is added to control urine (e.g. 40 ng/ml). The urine is then diluted 1:2, 1:4, 1:8 with normal urine.

Set up and label 15 (10 x 75 mm) glass test tubes. To tubes #1, 2, and 3, add 0.1 ml each of

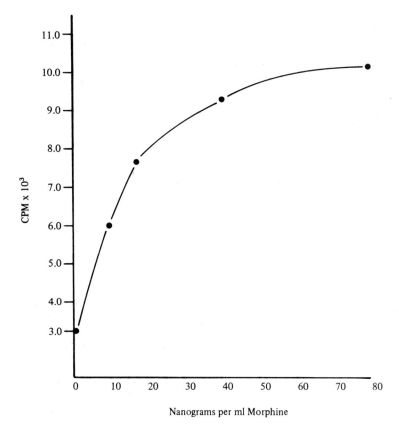

Nanograms per ml Morphine

FIGURE 4.

normal urine control; to tubes #4, 5, and 6, add 0.1 ml each of the 5 ng/ml morphine standard; to tubes #7, 8, and 9, add 0.1 ml each of the 10 ng/ml morphine standard; to tubes #10, 11, and 12, add 0.1 ml each of the 20 ng/ml morphine standard; and to tubes #13, 14, and 15, add 0.1 ml each of the 40 ng/ml standard. Proceed with steps 4 to 11 in the above protocol. A typical standard curve is shown as Figure 4.

Significant Facts Regarding Methodology

Tests Per Specimen and Controls

The number of tests made per patient specimen is left to the discretion of the user and his requirements. Because of the importance of control values in determinations, it is recommended that the positive control be processed in triplicate.

Specimens

Urine specimens do not require any special handling or pretreatment, but an effort should be made to keep pipetted samples free of gross debris.

Test Materials

Morphine is usually supplied as the soluble morphine sulfate; however, concentration should be expressed as weight of morphine per unit volume. Morphine test reagents will retain stability at ambient temperature and thus do not require refrigerated shipping; however, they should be kept under refrigeration (2 to 8°C) upon receipt. The reagents are stable for 4 months from date of manufacture.

Equipment

A centrifuge which generates 1,200 to 2,500 x g using swinging bucket rotor or 3,500 to 4,000 x g using a fixed angle head rotor may be used. The swinging bucket rotor is preferred because the pellet is formed at the bottom of the test tube and the supernatant is more easily removed than when the pellet is formed at an angle.

If a centrifuge with less gravitational force is used, centrifugation time must be extended until suitable pellets are formed.

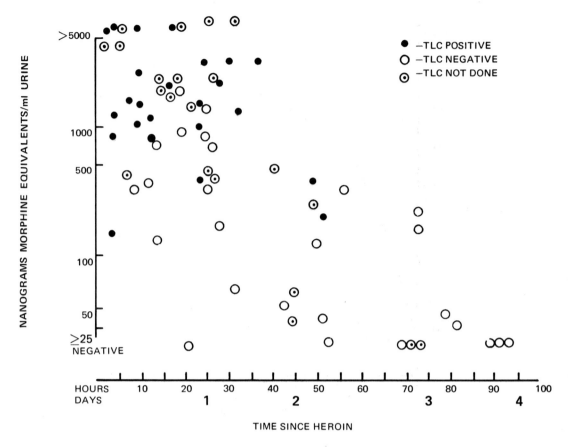

FIGURE 5.

Temperature Requirements

Ambient temperature is recommended throughout the procedure; temperature control is not critical at any step.

Timing

Incubation time should be no less than 10 min but can be extended to any time interval up to 24 hr. The time element is not critical. When incubation time is less than 1 hr, however, samples and standards must be incubated for the same period of time.

Time Study

The radioimmunoassay for morphine is not only highly sensitive, specific, and reliable, but fast and comparatively simple. A single test can be completed in approximately 30 min. Based on time studies run at Hoffman-La Roche, Inc., two technicians experienced in the ^{125}I-procedure can ideally process 1,050 samples in 7½ working hr, using the method described herein, while 1,250

samples can be processed using pre-mixed antibody and labeled antigen reagents. These procedures involved the use of manual equipment; the use of automatic pipetting technique has been evaluated and this can significantly increase the sample throughout.

Instrument Requirements

The most essential instrumentation requirement related to radioimmunoassay is for the quantification of radioactivity. Gamma counters are used for gamma energy-emitting isotopes, such as the more commonly used [125]I.

Manual systems are also commonly utilized in radioimmunoassays. This equipment has the disadvantages of not having automatic sample handling and data printout capabilities as well as having low counting efficiency. Liquid scintillation counters are required for counting beta energy-emitting isotopes such as tritium.

In addition to the above, the only other equipment commonly required is a centrifuge and pipetting equipment. The development of radio-immunoassay procedures for assays of drugs of abuse has intensified the already existing need for automation. The sample handling and reagent dispensing portion of radioimmunoassay procedures have been automated and automated counting equipment is found more and more frequently in laboratories.

Licensing

The levels of radioactivity contained in available individual radioimmunoassay kits utilizing ^{3}H as the isotope marker fall below the level at which licensing of the user by the U.S. Atomic Energy Commission is required. However, most kits utilizing ^{125}I, including those for morphine and barbiturates, are such that the user must hold either a general license obtainable through the AEC (form AEC-483), which "authorizes physicians, clinical laboratories and hospitals to possess certain ^{125}I in vitro clinical or laboratory tests," or a specific license that must be applied for through the AEC or an agreement state. Currently 23 of the 50 states are categorized as agreement states. Specific licenses are required by individuals who have need to use larger quantities than permitted under general license or who wish to use other isotopes.

Despite the need for licensing, the amounts of labeled material handled are such that reasonable laboratory care provides sufficient radiation protection. Disposal of radioactive wastes poses no serious problems, so that fear of using such materials is not well grounded.

RESULTS

The following studies were conducted on a double-blind basis and results indicate that, compared with available screening methods for the presence of morphine, the morphine radioimmunoassay provides high sensitivity (allowing a longer detection period), good specificity and notable reproducibility, making it an excellent diagnostic tool.

Study I

In the first study, the radioimmunoassay for morphine was evaluated for sensitivity and specificity, using urine from known heroin addicts, "normal" individuals and individuals receiving drugs other than heroin.[5] It involved urine samples collected from 94 patients applying for admission to a methadone clinic, 201 individuals classified as "normal" and 24 nonaddict patients known to be receiving specific drugs.

Of the 94 methadone clinic patients, 72 were reliably known to have used heroin within the past 96 hr. The concentration of morphine in urine samples from these 72 addicts, as determined by radioimmunoassay, is shown in Figure 5 as a function of time since heroin use. With one exception, the samples collected within 48 hr of estimated heroin use were found to contain more than 25 ng morphine equivalents per ml and a few samples were positive for as long as 78 hr.

Fifty of the above samples were also analyzed by TLC. Of the 50, only 24 (or 48%) were found positive for free morphine and none were shown positive after 48 hr. Radioimmunoassay showed that most of the samples found positive by TLC contained over 1,000 ng morphine equivalents per ml.

During the initial 24 hr, the most important time interval post-heroin use, radioimmunoassay failed to detect morphine equivalents in only 1 of the 43 samples taken, while TLC results were negative for 12 (or 40%) of 30 samples tested in the same interval. This comparison is also shown graphically in Figure 5. If the samples would have been hydrolyzed, the TLC results would be improved.

An additional 22 urine specimens were obtained from individuals attending the methadone clinic who were known not to have used heroin for at least one week and who were receiving orally at least 40 mg of methadone daily. All 22 specimens contained less than 25 ng morphine equivalents per ml. Of the 201 urines obtained from the "normal" population, 199 contained less than 25 ng/ml of morphine equivalents.

The study described here utilized a tritium label; re-evaluation of these studies with an iodine label, but the same antiserum lot, produced similar results except that the urines from volunteers receiving dextromethorphan showed significantly less or no cross-reactivity (25 ng/ml morphine equivalents).

Study II

In order to evaluate use of the assay in detecting morphine in serum, a study was run in which urine and serum samples were taken simultaneously from addict volunteers.[5] Figure 6 shows

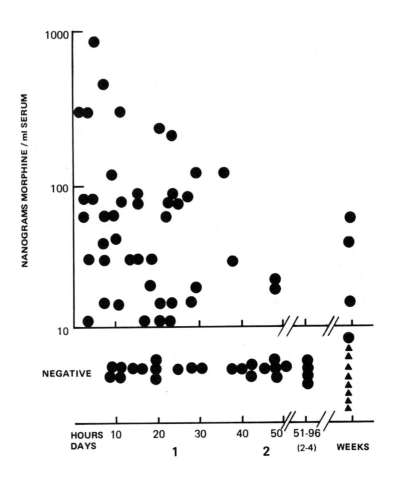

FIGURE 6.

the results of these values. The results would seem to indicate that the levels in serum are significantly lower than those found in urine. It appears that most addicts can be detected up to 12 hr after taking heroin and that between 12 and 50 hr after taking a heroin fix about 40% will be missed.

If the accuracy of the time when the heroin was taken is correct, it is also apparent that there is either a significant difference in the ability of people to metabolize and excrete heroin from the blood or that the results that appear negative are due to low doses of the narcotic. Since the addict has no way of knowing how much heroin he is taking, the latter is probably the most likely explanation for these results.

These data clearly indicate that urine specimens are preferable to serum for detection of heroin use.

Other clinical studies and comparisons of the radioimmunoassay technique with other methods are discussed elsewhere in this book.

Cross-reactivity

Employing a level of 25 ng morphine equivalents per ml as the cutoff point, no cross-reactivity was observed in the nonaddict patients taking standard doses of the following: oxymetazoline HCl, chloroquine, barbiturates, diphenhydramine HCL, phenylbutazone, caffeine, chlorpheniramine maleate, benztropine mesylate, prochlorperzine, propoxphene HCl, diphenylhydantoin, hydrochlorthiazide, glutethimide, amitriptyline HCl, chlordiazepoxide HCl, diphenoxylate HCl and atropine sulfate, thioridazine, meprobamate, chlorpheniramine maleate, phenylpropoanolaminide HCl and isopropamide, aminopyrine, methaqualone, trifluoperazine HCl, pentazocine, oxyphenbutazone, chlorpromazine, promethazine, and diazepam.

Also, four volunteers were given orally the maximal recommended dose of dextromethorphan contained in a commercial cough syrup every 6 hr for 4 days. During the 4-day medication period, 60 urine specimens from the 4 subjects were assayed and all had less than 40 ng morphine equivalents per ml.

Known Cross-reactants

The antiserum will react with levorotatory morphinans. The assay had positive results for up to 56 hr on urine specimens collected from an individual receiving 20 mg codeine orally in a prescription cough syrup. Codeine is recognized by the antibody as effectively as morphine. This is understandable in view of the fact that the carboxy group was placed in the 3 position and as a consequence the haptens used for conjugation of the surrogates of morphine are not recognized by the antibodies.

Relative reactivity was tested *in vitro* for morphine and its surrogates. The data developed in this study is included in the following table:

CONCLUSIONS

A radioimmunoassay has been developed to provide the needs for a reliable method of detection of heroin abuse. This assay has certain characteristics that offer advantages over other currently employed methodologies:

1. The extreme sensitivity of the RIA is advantageous at least in two ways; (a) a negative urine result is very strong evidence that clinically significant amounts of morphine or metabolites are not present and therefore additional analytical procedures are not necessary, and (b) morphine can be detected for longer periods of time than with less sensitive methods. It has the disadvantage that, because of reaction with similar molecules, each positive must be confirmed.

2. The results are totally objective with numerical values that eliminate the subjectivity of some of the other procedures.

3. The method for performing the assay is simple, not requiring hydrolysis of the urine. It measures total amount of drug present in the urine if it is sensitive to metabolites.

4. The test lends itself to automated procedures for high-speed processing if necessary.

Substance	Relative Detectability ($\mu g/ml$)
Morphine	0.1
Codeine	0.09
Morphine Glucuronide	0.125
Methadone	167
Meperidine	50
Dextromethorphan	100
Propoxyphene	1667
Nalorphine	167
Chlorpromazine	100
"Poppy Seeds"	500

REFERENCES

1. **Yalow, R. S. and Berson, S. A.,** Immunoassay of endogenous plasma insulin in man, *J. Clin. Invest.,* 39, 1157, 1960.
2. **Spector, S. and Parker, C. W.,** Morphine: radioimmunoassay, *Science,* 168, 1347, 1970.
3. **Spector, S., Berkowitz, B., Flynn, E. J., and Peskar, B.,** Anitbodies to morphine, barbiturates, and serotonin, *Pharmacol. Rev.,* 25, 281, 1973.
4. **Flynn, E. J. and Spector, S.,** Determinations of barbiturate derivatives by radioimmunoassay, *J. Pharmacol. Exp. Ther.,* 181, 547, 1972.
5. **Catlin, D., Cleeland, R., and Greenberg, E.,** A sensitive, rapid radioimmunoassay for morphine and immunologically related substances in urine and serum, *Clin. Chem.,* 19, 216, 1973.

USE OF THE DOUBLE ANTIBODY AND NITROCELLULOSE MEMBRANE FILTRATION TECHNIQUES TO SEPARATE FREE ANTIGEN FROM ANTIBODY BOUND ANTIGEN IN RADIOIMMUNOASSAYS

H. VanVunakis and L. Levine

TABLE OF CONTENTS

PRINCIPLE OF RADIOIMMUNOASSAY

Radioimmunoassays (RIA), originally applied to the measurement of insulin in plasma by Yalow and Berson,[1] today provide one of the most important techniques for the determination of biologically important molecules and their metabolites in physiological fluids. Among the desirable features possessed by RIA procedures are their specificity, sensitivity, and the rapidity with which the analysis can be carried out.

The principle of the technique can be expressed as follows:

$$Ag^* + Ab \rightleftarrows Ag^* \cdot Ab$$
$$+$$
$$Ag$$
$$\updownarrow$$
$$Ag \cdot Ab$$

Ag*   = free labeled antigen.
Ab   = antibody.
Ag   = free unlabeled antigen (in standard solutions or in sample to be analyzed).
Ag*·Ab = labeled antigen-antibody complex (bound antigen).

Labeled and unlabeled drugs compete for a limited number of antibody combining sites and the extent of the competition serves as a basis for the quantitative assay of the drug in test samples.

In the RIA technique, one must determine how much of the radioactive antigen is bound to antibody or how much is free. Separations of bound and free antigen have been achieved by a variety of procedures, including electrophoresis, chromatography, gel filtration, precipitation with reagents such as $(NH_4)_2SO_4$, adsorption to charcoal or other insoluble material or solid-phase antibodies, precipitation of the immune serum γ-globulin by a specific anti-γ-globulin, and filtration on nitrocellulose membranes. However, it is outside the purview of this report to describe all of these modifications. Instead, two specific modifications for measurement of combination of antigen with antibody will be presented. These are (1) the use of the double antibody technique to measure Ab-bound Ag and (2) the use of nitrocellulose membranes to measure Ab-bound Ag.

FACTORS GOVERNING ANTIGEN-ANTIBODY INTERACTIONS

Measurement of the combination of antibody with antigen is the objective of all serologic methods for quantitative estimation of antigen. Methods for measuring the interaction of multivalent antigen with antibody depend in part on the physical state of the reactants. These techniques and the principles behind them are covered in most textbooks of immunology.[2]

Many of the compounds with which we are concerned have only one combining site per molecule. Therefore, combination of antigen and antibody results in formation of soluble complexes, and must be treated as a reversible reaction. Their interaction with an antibody combining site can be expressed by the following equation:

$$Ag + Ab \rightleftarrows Ag \cdot Ab \qquad (1)$$

in which Ag represents the single combining site of the antigen (or drug) and Ab an antibody combining site. The association constant for the reaction is

$$\frac{[Ag \cdot Ab]}{[Ag][Ab]} = K. \qquad (2)$$

Under these conditions, if the combination of antibody with antigen is to be measured by physical separation of free and bound antigen, this separation must be accomplished by a procedure that minimizes perturbation of the equilibrium.

DOUBLE ANTIBODY TECHNIQUE

Principle

The specific antibody (Ab) is indistinguishable from other γ-globulin molecules in its antigenic properties. It retains these antigenic properties even when complexed with an antigen. Therefore, free Ag* remains in solution when the Ag* bound to the antibody (Ag* · Ab) is precipitated (along with the γ-globulin fraction) by anti-γ-globulin.

Long before the elucidation of the molecular structure of the antibody molecule, work from the laboratories of Landsteiner, Heidelberger, and Marrack among others had established that specific antibodies and normal γ-globulin preparations within a given species had common antigenic properties.[2] More recent studies of the antigenic properties of γ-globulins enable us to understand the molecular basis for these common antigenic properties.[3] It is clear that the conformations of the specific antibody in the absence and presence of the bound Ag (at least with an Ag composed of a single combining site) are indistinguishable and that their antigenic properties with respect to antibodies made in a foreign species are identical in the presence and absence of bound Ag. In addition, it is evident that their antigenic properties are identical with the corresponding class of normal immunoglobulins. The antigenic determinants common to the L-chains of all the immunoglobulin classes are also recognized by these antibodies produced in foreign species. Therefore, goat antisera to normal rabbit IgG, for example, contain antibodies that will not distinguish between normal rabbit IgG and specific rabbit antibodies of the IgG class. Furthermore, the goat antibodies will cross-react with rabbit immunoglobulins of all classes by virtue of common antigenic determinants in the L-chains.

These common antigenic properties are the basis of the double antibody technique since goat antibodies to rabbit γ-globulin will precipitate rabbit γ-globulin including the specific antibody being studied. Thus, in a reaction mixture in which an antigen of high specific activity is bound to its homologous antibody, addition of a goat anti-rabbit γ-globulin will precipitate the Ag only if it is bound to antibody. Obviously, for reasons of reproducibility and for maximum yield of bound Ag, conditions for precipitating all of the antibody must be used.

Procedure

As an example, a typical protocol and results of inhibition of [^{3}H] dihydromorphine anti-carboxymethylmorphine binding by morphine are shown in Table 1. The initial steps of the technique are carried out at room temperature. To a series of 10 X 75 mm No. 1 weight, light wall, disposable culture tubes are added in order: 0.1 ml diluent or 0.1 ml inhibitor serially diluted twofold or 0.1 ml unknown biological fluid suitably diluted, 0.1 ml radioactive antigen, and finally 0.1 ml of an immune serum dilution. An appropriate dilution of normal rabbit serum and the radioactive hapten serve as a control for nonspecific binding (tube 1). Binding is determined from the reaction mixture which contains an appropriate dilution of immune serum and the radioactive hapten (tube 2). After incubation at 37° for 1 hr, 0.1 ml of undiluted goat anti-rabbit γ-globulin is added and precipitation allowed to proceed at 2 to 4° for 16 to 18 hr. If the primary immune serum is used at a dilution of greater than 1:100, normal rabbit serum at a 1:100 dilution is added just prior to addition of the goat anti-rabbit γ-globulin. Care should be taken to mix the reaction contents after all additions, especially after addition of the rabbit immune serum and again after addition of the goat antiserum. The immune precipitates are collected by centrifugation at 1,500 X g for 30 min. The supernatant fluid is poured off with care and the tube, maintained in an inverted position, is placed in a rack lined with paper towels. If the tubes have been thoroughly cleaned in chromic acid cleaning solution, they will drain without forming channels. Without disturbing the precipitate, the sides of the tubes above the precipitate are wiped carefully with strips of Whatman® No. 1 filter paper. The precipitate is dissolved in 0.2 ml 0.1 N NaOH and transferred to scintillation vials for radioactive analysis. If the antigen has been labeled with radioactive iodine rather than ^{3}H or ^{14}C, the tube containing the precipitate is counted directly.

Factors to be Considered When Setting Up the Technique

A schematic representation of an antigen-antibody precipitin curve separated into regions of antibody excess, equivalence, and antigen excess is shown in Figure 1. In this precipitin reaction, the antigen is rabbit γ-globulin, while the antibody (anti-γ-globulin) was produced in a goat following immunization with rabbit γ-globulin. The amount of antigen precipitated by a constant amount of antiserum depends upon the amount of the antigen added. Of importance is the fact that in the region of antibody excess and in the equivalence zone all of the rabbit γ-globulin is precipitated. The presence of additional amounts of rabbit γ-globulin limits lattice formation of antigen-antibody intermediates and results in a smaller precipitate. All of the rabbit γ-globulin is not precipitated in this region of antigen excess. Therefore, in order to separate free Ag* from Ag* · Ab quantitatively, one must use sufficient goat anti-γ-globulin to precipitate all of the rabbit γ-globulin (i.e., one must work in the zones of equivalence or antibody excess).

When the titers of specific antibody are high, the amount of γ-globulin (the antigen in this double antibody procedure) in the diluted antisera may not be sufficient to form a precipitate with enough bulk to permit its collection in a quantitative manner. A uniform amount of rabbit γ-globulin (usually in the form of a dilution of normal rabbit sera) is added for the purpose of maintaining the uniformity of the immune precipitate. For quantitative recovery of Ag* · Ab, the system should be in antibody excess with respect to the goat anti-rabbit γ-globulin.

Advantages of the Double Antibody Technique

As mentioned previously, separation of Ab-

TABLE 1

Inhibition of [³H] Dihydromorphine Anti-carboxymethylmorphine Binding by Morphine

Reaction mixture:	1	2	3	4	5	6	7	8
Ml isotris buffer	0.1	0.1	—	—	—	—	—	—
Ml inhibitor, morphine, serially diluted	—	—	0.1	0.1	0.1	0.1	0.1	0.1
Ng inhibitor, morphine, added	—	—	1.0	0.5	0.25	0.125	0.062	0.031
Ml [³H] dihydromorphine 13,500 cpm/0.1 ml	0.1	0.1	0.1	0.1	0.1	0.1	0.1	0.1
Ml normal rabbit serum (1:100)	0.1	—	—	—	—	—	—	—
Ml rabbit anti-morphine (1:100)	—	0.1	0.1	0.1	0.1	0.1	0.1	0.1
			Incubate at 37° for 60 min					
Ml normal rabbit serum* (1:100)	0.1	0.1	0.1	0.1	0.1	0.1	0.1	0.1
Ml goat anti-rabbit γ-globulin, undiluted	0.1	0.1	0.1	0.1	0.1	0.1	0.1	0.1
			Incubate at 2 to 4° Overnight					
Cpm in precipitate	476	5,977	1,532	2,250	3,080	3,902	4,762	5,632
	485	5,785	1,604	2,163	3,216	3,763	4,792	5,408
	463	6,125	1,583	2,342	3,162	3,840	4,931	5,392
Percent Inhibition	—	—	80	68	51	39	21	9

*If the immune serum is used at a dilution >1:100, 0.1 ml normal rabbit serum at a dilution of 1:100 should be added here.

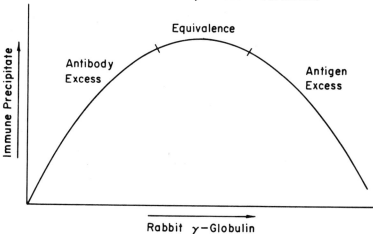

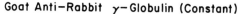

Goat Anti−Rabbit γ−Globulin (Constant)

FIGURE 1. Schematic representation of a quantitative precipitin reaction between rabbit γ-globulin and goat antibody to rabbit γ-globulin.

bound Ag from free Ag should not perturb the equilibrium shown in reaction [2]. In the double antibody procedure, the specific antibody being multivalent is rapidly "surrounded" by many anti-γ-globulin molecules and a soluble lattice is formed. This soluble lattice composed of Ag* · Ab anti-γ-globulin complexes tends to prevent dissociation of the Ag* from the Ag* · Ab combination trapped in the lattice. Therefore, addition of a potent anti-γ-globulin solution may "freeze" the Ag* bound in the Ag* · Ab form.

The technique has been used for many different substances since it was first adapted for use in the RIA of hormones.[4,5] Some of the immune systems that have been characterized in our laboratory and for which RIA's have been developed are listed in Table 2. Most of these antisera were produced in rabbits but a few were made by immunizing guinea pigs and monkeys. When antisera are produced in guinea pigs or monkeys, rabbit anti-guinea pig γ-globulin and rabbit anti-monkey-γ-globulin may be used as the precipitating antibody. Many of these antigens have properties for which several separation procedures could be used, e.g., morphine, ammonium sulfate precipitation,[6] and nitrocellulose membrane filtration.[7] However, each of these separation techniques has its own peculiarities and a procedure that separates antigen X in the free and antibody-bound form may not separate antigen Y in its free and bound forms. A technician who has mastered

the double antibody technique can perform all RIA's, whether the antigen be a small molecular weight substance, such as a drug, or a macromolecule, such as protein[4,5] or DNA.[8]

Disadvantages of the Double Antibody Techniques

The two major disadvantages of the double antibody procedure which are considerable when discussing a mass scanning technique for use in measurement of drugs are (1) the number of steps in the procedure, for example, addition of Ag, Ab, carrier γ-globulin, second Ab, followed by centrifugation, and analysis of the precipitate or supernatant fluid to quantitate the amount of label in the fraction and (2) the length of time required for precipitation. Although the rates of the initial molecular antigen-antibody reactions, which lead to formation of soluble lattices and eventually precipitates, are diffusion controlled, the formation of a lattice large enough for precipitation is relatively slow. Therefore, for precipitation sufficient for quantitative analysis, incubation from 10 to 20 hr at 2 to 4° may be required.

If the physiological fluid to be assayed is sera or plasma, the γ-globulin in these fluids may cross-react with the goat anti-γ-globulin, thus diminishing the amount of goat antibody available to form immune precipitate with the rabbit γ-globulin. The system may be pushed into antigen excess (Figure 1), thus decreasing the amount of Ag* · Ab in the immune precipitate. In such cases, the amounts of

TABLE 2

Some Immune Systems Characterized in This Laboratory in which Ag* · Ab Was Separated from Ag* by Precipitation of the Immune Serum γ-Globulin with a Specific Anti-γ-Globulin

Compound	Labeled antigen
Morphine	[^{3}H]-Dihydromorphine
	[^{125}I]-Copolymer-carboxymethylmorphine
D-LSD	[^{3}H]-LSD
	[^{125}I]-Copolymer-lysergamide
3,4,5-Trimethoxyphen-	[^{125}I]-N-(3',4',5'-Trimethoxyphen-
ethylamine (mescaline)	ethyl)-4-hydroxy-phenylacetamide
	[^{125}I]-Copolymer-mescaline
THC	[^{125}I]-Copolymer-carboxymethyl-THC
Nicotine	[^{3}H]-Nicotine
Cotinine	[^{125}I]-N-(p-Hydroxyphenethyl)-trans-
	4'-cotinine-carboxamide
3,4-Dimethoxyphenethyl-	[^{125}I]-N-(3',4'-Dimethoxyphenethyl)-
amine (DMPEA)	4-hydroxy-phenylacetamide
	[^{125}I]-Copolymer-DMPEA
Normetanephrine	[^{125}I]-Copolymer-normetanephrine
Several prostaglandins	[^{3}H]-Prostaglandins
and their metabolites	[^{125}I]-Copolymer-prostaglandins
Pseudouridine	[^{14}C]-Pseudouridine
7-Methylguanosine	[^{3}H]-7-Methylguanosine
N^2-Methylguanosine	[^{3}H]-N^2-Methylguanosine
N^2-Dimethylguanosine	[^{3}H]-N^2-Dimethylguanosine
Human serum albumin	[^{125}I]-human serum albumin
S100 protein	[^{125}I]-S100 protein
UV-irradiated DNA	[^{125}I]-UV-irradiated DNA

fluids analyzed should be kept constant and additional goat antisera should be added if needed to assure that the immune precipitate would be formed in antibody excess.

There are also reports in the literature that complement components may interfere with this assay.[9] EDTA added to the buffer can overcome such difficulties. For use in drug scanning, such potential interfering materials, as cross-reacting γ-globulin in the biological fluid being analyzed or the presence of complement which may decrease the rate of precipitation, can be eliminated from consideration if the durgs are extracted from blood or tissues before RIA. In urine, γ-globulin or complement ordinarily would not be present.

Anti-γ-globulin sera, in the amounts required to form the immune precipitate, can be expensive if purchased from commercial sources. The cost of this reagent diminishes greatly if the experimenter has access to a large animal species which can be immunized with the appropriate γ-globulin.

LABELED HAPTENS

As we have discussed above, RIA depends on the competition of labeled and unlabeled antigen for antibody. The sensitivity of the assay in detecting haptens in biological fluids depends in part upon the specific activity of the labeled hapten. Haptens cannot always be labeled by synthetic routes or by exchange reactions to specific activities sufficiently high to be useful in competitive binding assays. However, it is often possible to chemically modify a hapten to permit reaction with radioactive iodine[10] by coupling the hapten (or a functionalized derivative) to a protein[11] or copolymer[12] containing tyrosine or to a tyrosine derivative.[13]

Multivalent Hapten

The multivalent antigen has been particularly useful in developing an RIA for tetrahydrocannabinol. With the antisera of rabbits immunized with carboxymethyl THC, after quantitative precipitation of the rabbit antibody with goat anti-rabbit γ-globulin, we could not detect binding of ^{14}C or [3]H Δ^9THC, 11-OH-Δ^8THC, or 8,11-diOH-Δ^9THC (provided by the National Institute of Mental Health with specific activities between 17 and 25 $\mu c/mg$). However, binding of an [125]I *multivalent* THC antigen to antibody was detected after separation of bound antigen by the double antibody technique (Figure 2A). The specificities of the antisera were determined by comparing the inhibiting capacities of several cannabinoid derivatives (Figure 2B and Table 3). The antisera do not differentiate the position of the double bond in Δ^8THC and Δ^9THC since both of these compounds are equally good inhibitors of the reaction. The additional hydroxyl group in 11-OH-Δ^8THC is also not recognized by the antibodies. Cannabinol (which is a dibenzo-pyran) reacts somewhat less effectively. Cannabidiol with an open pyran ring but with the remaining structure similar to Δ^9THC gives very low inhibition at best. Cannabicyclol which possesses a bicyclic terpene moiety is not inhibitory.

From the limited number of cannabinoid derivatives available for this study, it appears that the antibodies recognize the tetrahydrocannabinol and cannabinol structures and can be used to estimate the net content of Δ^9THC, Δ^8THC, 11-OH-Δ^9THC, and cannabinol without interference from cannabinoid derivatives with greater diversity of structure. The antigen-antibody reaction is inhibited from 39 to 54% by 10 ng of Δ^8THC, Δ^9THC, and 11-OH-Δ^8THC.

In addition to obtaining an antigen of relatively high specific activity, another advantage in employing a multivalent antigen capable of forming an antigen-antibody lattice is that nonspecific forces present in lattice-forming antigen-antibody reactions will amplify specific hapten-antibody forces and facilitate measurement of bound hapten, especially in immune systems with low affinity. The amplification of measurable binding by the multivalent antigen has been noticed in several systems.[14] For example, when multivalent ^{125}I-copoly-lysergamide conjugate[15] or

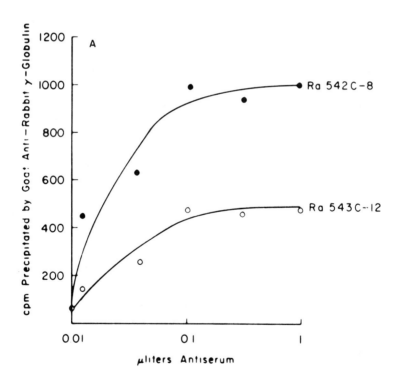

FIGURE 2A. Binding of [^{125}I]-carboxymethyl THC-copolymer by rabbit anti-THC. The labeled carboxymethyl THC-copolymer, approximately 15,000 cpm per reaction mixture, was incubated with the antisera in a 0.3 ml reaction volume for 1 hr at 37°. Following addition of carrier rabbit γ-globulin in a 0.1 ml volume, goat anti-rabbit γ-globulin (0.1 ml) was added and immune precipitation was allowed to proceed overnight at 2 to 4°; about 100 cpm were precipitated in the presence of normal rabbit serum.

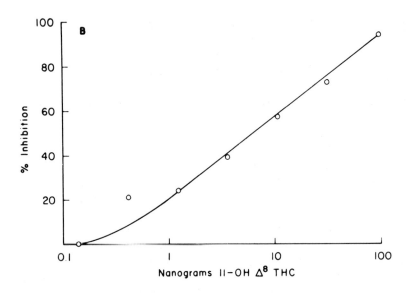

FIGURE 2B. Inhibition of the [^{125}I]-carboxymethyl THC-copolymer anti-THC binding by varying amounts of 11-OH-Δ^8THC. Experimental conditions same as those described in Figure 2A.

[^{3}H] D-LSD was incubated with rabbit anti-lysergamide under identical conditions and the antigen-antibody complexes precipitated by goat anti-rabbit γ-globulin, it was found that 10% of the [^{3}H] LSD was precipitated by a 1/200 dilution of antiserum whereas 10% of the multivalent antigen was precipitated with a 1/2,000 dilution of the same antiserum. Comparison of specificities of the antigen-antibody reactions when measured with multivalent copolymer conjugates and monovalent antigen using the same antiserum indicates that the specificities are qualitatively similar.

TABLE 3

Inhibition of the Binding Between [^{125}I] THC-Copolymer and Anti-THC by Cannabinoids

	Antisera			
	(Ra 542C-8) inhibition		(Ra 543C-12) inhibition	
Compound	100 ng	10 ng	100 ng	10 ng
	%	%	%	%
Δ^9 THC	69	39	43	20
Δ^8 THC	76	45	32	11
11-OH-Δ^8 THC	82	54	37	27
Cannabinol	53	23	24	13
Cannabicyclol	10	0	5	3
Cannabidiol	0	0	6	0

One disadvantage of using the multivalent antigen is that, for the reasons already discussed, unlabeled monovalent hapten cannot compete as effectively as the labeled multivalent hapten for the limited number of antibody sites. Other reasons for unfavorable competition may also exist. For example, some antibodies recognize not only the hapten but the covalent link formed between the hapten and the carrier molecule during the synthesis of the immunizing conjugates. Since the multivalent antigen contains the entire antigenic determinant, that is, the hapten as well as the link to the carrier, it competes much more effectively for such antibodies than the monovalent hapten which has not been appropriately derivatized. Binding of a labeled hapten which lacks the link represents a cross-reaction with such an antibody. Since the cross-reaction would have less of an association constant, it would be easier to inhibit with the hapten as it exists in biological fluids. Therefore, a labeled monovalent antigen of sufficiently high specific activity, if available, may be more useful.

Monovalent Hapten

In the case of mescaline, antibodies were produced in rabbits immunized with conjugates formed by coupling mescaline to human serum albumin by the use of carbodiimide. For this RIA, a monovalent derivative, N-(3',4',5'-trimethoxy-

TABLE 4

Inhibition by Mescaline and Related Compounds of the
$[^{125}I]$ N-(3',4',5' Trimethoxyphenethyl)-4-Hydroxy-
phenylacetamide-anti-mescaline Reaction

Compound	Nmol required for 50% inhibition
	Ra 644
3,4,5-Trimethoxyphenetic acid (mescaline)	0.012
N-methyl-3,4,5-trimethoxy-phenethylamine	0.013
3,4,5-Trimethoxyphenylacetamine	1.46
2,3,4-Trimethoxyphenethylamine	41.0
3,4-Dimethoxyphenethylamine	48
3,5-Dimethoxyphenylethylamine	370
3-Methoxy-4-hydroxyphenethylamine	>280*

Reaction conditions: $[^{125}I]$ mescaline derivative (11,000 cpm) was incubated with a 1/100
dilution of antibody and increments of each
inhibitor in a volume of 0.3 ml for 60 min at 37°.
A 0.1-ml aliquot of undiluted goat anti-rabbit
γ-globulin (titered to be in antibody excess) was
added and the reaction mixture was incubated
overnight at 2 to 4°. After centrifugation, the
immune precipitate containing Ag* · Ab was
counted in a Packard auto-gamma spectrometer.
Approximately 170 cpm were precipitated in the
absence of the immune serum.

*Less than 10% at this level.

---

phenethyl)4-hydroxyphenylacetamide, was
synthesized and labeled with ^{125}I to a specific
activity of 100 $\mu c/\mu g$. As shown in Table 4, 50%
inhibition of the antigen-antibody reaction is
obtained with 0.012 nmol of mescaline; as little as
300 pg of mescaline can be measured with this
assay.[16]

The antibodies to mescaline are sensitive both
to the number and position of the methoxyl
substitutions. The 2,3,4-trimethoxyphenethyla-
mine derivative is 3,000 times less effective than
mescaline in inhibiting the antigen-antibody reaction. Dimethoxy and monomethoxyphenethyla-
mine are even less inhibitory. Dopamine and
normetanephrine give less than 10% inhibition at
the 250 nmol level. This antiserum is much less sensitive to structural changes in the side chain, e.g.,
N-methyl mescaline is an equally effective inhibi-

tor, while the acid metabolite (3,4,5-trimethoxy-
phenethylacetic acid) is one-hundreth as effective.

NITROCELLULOSE MEMBRANE TECHNIQUE

Principle

This modification utilizes the binding properties of nitrocellulose membranes, i.e., affinity for
protein, and microfiltration, to separate Ag* · Ab
complexes from free Ag*. The technique is applicable to Ag*–Ab systems in which the Ag* itself
does not bind to the filter.

Procedure

Primary immune binding and inhibition of
immune binding in the double antibody and
nitrocellulose membrane filtration techniques are
performed identically. Analysis of bound hapten is
different. As an example, a typical protocol and
results of inhibition of $[^3H]$ dihydromorphine
anti-carboxymethylmorphine binding by codeine
are shown in Table 5.

To a series of acid-washed, disposable culture
tubes (10 X 75 mm No. 1 weight, light wall) are
added in the following order: 0.1 ml diluent or 0.1
ml inhibitor serially diluted twofold or 0.1 ml
unknown biological fluid suitably diluted; 0.1 ml
radioactive antigen; and finally 0.1 ml of an
immune serum dilution. An appropriate dilution
of normal rabbit serum and the radioactive hapten
source serve as a control for nonspecific binding.

After incubation at 37° for 30 min, 1 ml of
buffer is added to a reaction mixture. After
mixing, the contents of the tube are transferred
with a Pasteur pipette to the filter pad and the
liquid removed by suction. The filter well is
washed with about 10 ml buffer. In our laboratory, transfer of 30 samples is accomplished in
about 15 min using a commercially available
manifold. The filters are transferred to scintillation
vials and counted for radioactivity.

Factors to Be Considered When Setting Up the Technique

As mentioned before, rates of combination
between antigen and antibody are extremely fast.
They approach the theoretical limit of 10^9 1
mol^{-1} sec^{-1} for diffusion-limited reactions. In
RIA's of monovalent antigens, the time for the
analysis of bound and free antigen is the main
limitation. Therefore, for drug screening a simple

TABLE 5

Inhibition of $[^3H]$ Dihydromorphine Anti-morphine Binding by Codeine

Reaction mixture:	1	2	3	4	5	6	7	8	9
Ml isotris buffer	0.1	0.1	–	–	–	–	–	–	–
Ml codeine, serially diluted	–	–	0.1	0.1	0.1	0.1	0.1	0.1	0.1
Ng codeine; 0.1 ml	–	–	1.0	0.5	0.25	0.12	0.06	0.03	0.015
Ml $[^3H]$ dihydromorphine 7,000 cpm/0.1 ml	0.1	0.1	0.1	0.1	0.1	0.1	0.1	0.1	0.1
Ml normal rabbit serum (1:500)	0.1	–	–	–	–	–	–	–	–
Ml rabbit anti-morphine (1:500)	–	0.1	0.1	0.1	0.1	0.1	0.1	0.1	0.1
			Incubate at 37° for 30 min						
			Add 1 ml of buffer and filter						
Cpm on filter	250 300	1,915 1,992	478 523	584 587	838 851	1,032 981	1,423 1,336	1,772 1,724	1,932 2,087
Percent Inhibition			87	82	66	56	34	12	0

procedure like filtration, which immediately separates antibody-bound from free antigen, has advantages over the more general double antibody procedure which depends upon the relatively slow formation of the immune precipitate.

Binding of antibody-bound antigen by nitrocellulose membranes should reflect the combination of antigen to antibody. The reference procedure for measuring the combination of small molecules with antibodies is equilibrium dialysis. Therefore, the combination of [^{3}H]dihydromorphine with anti-3-carboxymethylmorphine was measured by estimating antibody-bound [^{3}H]dihydromorphine by equilibrium dialysis and by filtration through nitrocellulose membranes. Average association constants of 1.08×10^8 l mol^{-1} and 8.3×10^7 l mol^{-1} were calculated from the data obtained at 2 to 4° by filtration and by equilibrium dialysis, respectively. An average association constant of 2×10^7 l mol^{-1} at 34° was obtained by calculation of binding data obtained by filtration through nitrocellulose membranes.

The rates of binding of 1 pmol [^{3}H]dihydromorphine with our antiserum to morphine at 0 and 37°, respectively, are extremely rapid. Even at 0°, the reaction is over in 1 min, at the concentrations of antigen and antisera used in the RIA. Therefore, time of the initial reaction is not a factor in development of a rapid assay for morphine and most likely other drugs of abuse. The binding of [^{3}H]dihydromorphine to anti-3-carboxymethylmorphine, as measured by filtration through nitrocellulose membranes, is shown in Figure 3A. With one μl of antiserum the binding approached 50%. At higher concentrations of antiserum, the amount of hapten-antibody complex bound to the filter was even greater. Inhibition of the dihydromorphine anti-3-carboxymethylmorphine reaction by morphine, codeine, dihydrocodeine, and heroin is shown in Figure 3B.[7]

Morphine is still easily detectable in the urine of the mouse 40 hr after intraperitoneal administration of 500 μg. Morphine or heroin can easily be detected at the 10-ng level in blood without the prior extraction of the serum. This filter, 25 mm diameter, retains about 700 μg of serum proteins before its binding capacity is exceeded; therefore, the reaction mixtures should contain <10 μl of undiluted serum. Morphine or heroin in blood or urine at pg levels, however, would have to be measured after extraction.

Advantages of the Nitrocellulose Membrane Filtration Technique

The procedure is simple, rapid, and precise. Even without automated instrumentation, one technician can routinely analyze 100 samples within 3 hr. With the proper instrumentation it could be adapted to laboratories that do mass screening.

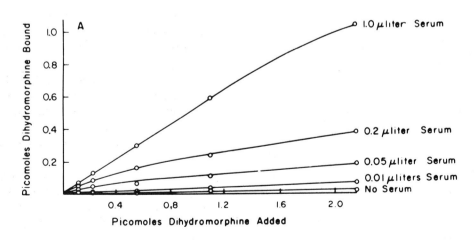

FIGURE 3A. Binding of [^{3}H]dihydromorphine to anti-3-carboxymethylmorphine. The indicated amounts of [^{3}H]dihydromorphine and anti-3-carboxymethylmorphine antiserum were incubated at 37° for 30 min in a total volume of 0.3 ml and then filtered through nitrocellulose membranes. The filters were dried and counted for radioactivity. Each point is the mean of two determinations.

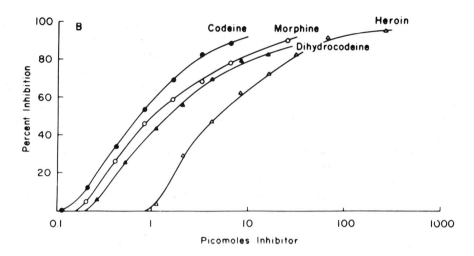

FIGURE 3B. Inhibition of dihydromorphine binding to anti-3-carboxymethylmorphine by morphine, codeine, heroin, and dihydrocodeine. [^{3}H]dihydromorphine (1.05 pmol) plus the indicated amounts of nonradioactive inhibitor was mixed in a total volume of 0.3 ml. The reaction was started by the addition of 0.1 ml of a 1:500 dilution of anti-3-carboxymethylmorphine (0.2 μl) and incubated at 37° for 30 min. The reaction mixtures were filtered and the filters dried and counted for radioactivity in a liquid scintillation counter. Each point is the mean of at least two determinations. Data from Gershman et al.[7]

Disadvantages of the Nitrocellulose Membrane Filtration Technique

The technique is applicable only to hapten-antibody systems in which the hapten does not bind to the nitrocellulose filter. However, continual progress is being made by industry in developing filters of different compositions and pore sizes for various microfiltration problems. Such filters might be useful with haptens that bind to nitrocellulose membranes.

USE OF SPECIFIC ANTIBODIES AND NATURALLY OCCURRING RECEPTORS IN COMPETITIVE BINDING ASSAYS

It is now possible to assay several compounds of biological interest by competitive binding procedures using either an antibody prepared in an experimental animal or a naturally occurring molecule such as a tissue receptor or a binding protein of blood.[17] For example, sensitive assays for cyclic AMP have been developed using antibodies[18] and intracellular receptors.[19] The specificity of the natural receptor may or may not be as narrow as an antibody. The organic chemist has the advantage over nature in that he can produce antibodies in experimental animals that recognize different structural features of a molecule. On the other hand, for some compounds such as the catecholamines, antibodies suitable for sensitive RIA's have not been produced despite attempts made in several laboratories. A receptor binding assay for norepinephrine using a protein solubilized from a microsomal fraction of canine ventricular myocardium has recently been described.[20]

It is the availability, stability, and solubility of the tissue receptors which pose, perhaps, the greatest problem in the use of the receptor macromolecules for assay purposes. Recently, characterization and localization of LSD[21] and opiate receptors[22,23] in subcellular fractions of nervous tissue have been reported. In the case of LSD receptors, high affinity binding sites on the synaptosomal membrane from rat cerebral cortical gray matter are present in extremely small amounts and do in some respects have a specificity similar to that of the antibody.[15] These sites have still to be solubilized from the synaptosomal membrane.

Not every physiological receptor will provide a practical alternative to antibodies in developing assay procedures for compounds of neurochemical interest. However, information of drug-receptor site interactions on the molecular level is basic to the understanding of the drug's action in vivo. Such studies also furnish information about the conformations that related molecules might possess in solution (or may have induced upon them by virtue of their binding to these receptors), which may be valuable in designing structural analogues of the drug which would effectively occupy the site and perhaps prevent the drug from exerting its biological effects. (In vivo studies would of course reveal whether an analogue meets the other requirements, e.g., ability to pass the blood brain barrier and survive metabolic inactivation.)

REFERENCES

1. Yalow, R. S. and Berson, S. A., Immunoassay of endogenous plasma insulin in man, *J. Clin. Invest.*, 39, 1157, 1960.
2. Kabat, E. A. and Mayer, M. M., *Experimental Immunochemistry*, Charles C Thomas, Springfield, Ill., 1961.
3. Kabat, E. A., *Structural Concepts in Immunology and Immunochemistry*, Holt, Rinehart and Winston, New York, 1968.
4. Utiger, R. D., Parker, M. L., and Daughaday, W. H., Studies on human growth hormone. I. A radioimmunoassay for human growth hormone, *J. Clin. Invest.*, 41, 254, 1962.
5. Morgan, C. R. and Lazarow, A., Immunoassay of insulin – plasma insulin levels of normal subdiabetic and diabetic rats, *Diabetes*, 12, 115, 1963.
6. Spector, S. and Parker, C. W., Morphine: Radioimmunoassay, *Science*, 168, 1347, 1970.
7. Gershman, H., Powers, E., Levine, L., and Van Vunakis, H., Radioimmunoassay of prostaglandins, angiotensin, digoxin, morphine, and adenosine-3',5'-cyclic'-monophosphate with nitrocellulose membranes, *Prostaglandins*, 1, 407, 1972.
8. Seamen, E., Van Vunakis, H., and Levine, L., Serologic estimation of thymine dimers in the DNA of bacterial and mammalian cells following irradiation with ultraviolet light and postirradiation repair, *J. Biol. Chem.*, 247, 5709, 1972.
9. Daughaday, W. H. and Jacobs, L. S., Methods of separating antibody-bound from free antigen, in *Principles of Competitive Protein-Binding Assays*, Odell, W. D. and Daughaday, W. H., Eds., Lippincott, Philadelphia, 1971.
10. Hunter, W., The preparation of radioiodinated proteins of high specific activity, their reaction with antibody *in vitro*: The radioimmunoassay, in *Handbook of Experimental Immunology*, Weir, D. M., Ed., Blackwell, Oxford, 1967, 608.
11. Rees Midgley, A., Jr., Niswender, G. D., and Sri Ram, J., Haptenradioimmunoassay: A general procedure for the estimation of steroidal and other haptenic substances, *Steroids*, 13, 731, 1969.
12. Newton, W. T., McGuigan, J. E., and Jaffe, B. M., Radioimmunoassay of peptides lacking tyrosine, *J. Lab. Clin. Med.*, 75, 886, 1970.
13. Goodfriend, T. L. and Ball, D. L., Radioimmunoassay of bradykinin: Chemical modification to enable use of radioactive iodine, *J. Lab. Clin. Med.*, 73, 501, 1969.
14. Levine, L., Gutierrez Cernosek, R. M., Polet, H., and Gershman, H., Prostaglandins: Serologic specificities and estimation in biological fluids, in *Third Conference on Prostaglandins in Fertility Control*, Bergström, S., Green, K., and Samuelsson, B., Eds., W.H.O. Research and Training Centre on Human Reproduction, Karolinska Institutet, Stockholm, 1972, 38.
15. Van Vunakis, H., Farrow, J. T., Gjika, H. B., and Levine, L., Specificity of the antibody receptor site to D-lysergamide: model of a physiological receptor for lysergic acid diethylamide, *Proc. Natl. Acad. Sci.*, 68, 1483, 1971.
16. Riceberg, L. and Van Vunakis, H., Radioimmunoassay for mescaline, in preparation.
17. Odell, W. D. and Daughaday, W. H., Eds., *Principles of Competitive Protein-Binding Assays*, Lippincott, Philadelphia, 1971.
18. Steiner, A. L., Kipnis, D. M., Utiger, R., and Parker, C., Radioimmunoassay for the measurement of adenosine 3',5'-cyclic phosphate, *Proc. Natl. Acad. Sci.*, 367, 1969.
19. Gilman, A. G., A protein binding assay for adenosine 3'5'-cyclic monophosphate, *Proc. Natl. Acad. Sci.*, 67, 305, 1970.
20. Lefkowitz, R. J., Haber, E., and O'Hara, D., Identification of the cardiac beta-adrenergic receptor protein: Solubilization and purification by affinity chromatography, *Proc. Natl. Acad. Sci.*, 69, 2828, 1972.
21. Farrow, J. T. and Van Vunikas, H., Characteristics of D-lysergic acid diethylamide binding to subcellular fractions derived from rat brain, *Biochem. Pharmacol.*, 22, 1103, 1973.
22. Pert, C. B. and Snyder, S. H., Opiate receptor: Demonstration in nervous tissue, *Science*, 179, 1011, 1973.
23. Simon, E. J., The current status of the morphine receptor, *Fed. Proc.*, in press.

DRUG TESTING BY HEMAGGLUTINATION-INHIBITION*

F. L. Adler

TABLE OF CONTENTS

INTRODUCTION

The recent development of serological techniques for the detection of commonly abused drugs has provided rapid and highly sensitive diagnostic test procedures. In view of the pressures for drug testing on an ever-increasing scale, many of these methods have found their way into toxicological laboratories with little but the promotional literature for backing. Therefore, it is not surprising that confusion exists with regard to the proper use and interpretation of the serological tests and their relation to the more conventional chromatographic and fluorometric procedures. The far-reaching consequences of a false diagnosis of drug abuse demand that those engaged in testing not only master the arts of the various techniques but that they also be fully informed about basic principles, limitations, and appropriate interpretations. While this presentation will concern itself primarily with one serological test, namely hemagglutination-inhibition (HI) a more general consideration of serological testing appears unavoidable in view of that which has just been discussed.

Immunochemical studies of the past 50 years, particularly the work of Landsteiner,[1] have shown that antibodies reactive to substances of low molecular weight can be produced by immunization of animals with conjugates of such substances (haptens) to fully immunogenic proteins (carriers). A summary of methods applicable to the synthesis of a wide variety of such conjugates has been published.[2] Of special relevance to the topic to be discussed is the general recognition that only some of the antibodies produced in this manner are specific for the hapten and that this specificity, although often great, is not absolute.

THEORETICAL CONSIDERATIONS

The immunologist's concept of specificity often appears to be at variance with that of the toxicologist. While the latter is concerned with the methods that identify a given drug or a particular metabolite of a drug, the immunologist deals with the detection of the binding of antibodies by antigenic determinants. Such determinants may and do occur not only in the pharmacologically active drug but also in closely related substances, including some of the metabolites. The maximal size of determinants has been operationally defined for some proteins where it corresponds to the space occupied by a folded peptide of 5 to 8 amino acid residues; the minimal size remains to be clearly established. The data presented in Table 1 illustrate this point by showing that consumers of poppy seeds excrete substances in their urine which react with antibodies produced in response to morphine conjugates in a

*This work was supported in part by Grant DA-00120 from the National Institute of Mental Health, and by Contract DADA17-72C-2052, Department of Army, U.S. Army Medical Research and Development Command, Washington, D.C.

TABLE 1

False Positive Test for Morphine After Ingestion of Poppy Seeds

Subject	Dose (X)	Morphine equivalents μg/ml urine
FA	3[a]	2.5–5.0
DC	2	1.3
IK	1	0.3
SB	1	0.6
UA	1	0.3
LA	1	0.3

[a]Number of pieces of pastry containing poppy seed filling eaten.

TABLE 2

Inhibitory Activity of Glucuronide Bound Morphine

Rabbit	Serum dil.	Inhibition titer of morphine glucuronide		Inhib. by morphine (ng/ml)	Bound/free
		Not hydrolyzed	Hydrolyzed		
181	100	800	800	6–12	1:1
	200	1,600	1,600		1:1
	400	3,200–6,400	3,200–6,400		1:1
437	800	50	800	3–6	1:16
	1,600	200	1,600–3,200		1:16
	3,200	400–800	>6,400		
456	4,000	50	400–800	6	1:8–1:16
	8,000	100	1,000		1:16
487	2,000	50–100	200–400	3–6	1:4
	4,000	200	800–1,600		1:4–1:8
	8,000	400	1,600–3,200		1:4–1:8

Note: The morphine-glucuronide preparation was purified and free of morphine detectable by TLC.

manner which renders these gourmets indistinguishable from heroin addicts. It is likely that in future work, either through appropriate absorption of the antisera or by selection of alternate "specific" conjugates, more selective antibodies may be produced or selected and that such reagents may no longer react with poppy seed extracts or with dextromethorphan, to name but two examples. However, it seems most unlikely that antibodies reactive with morphine and with morphine alone will be produced. Not only would this tax the rabbit's discriminatory ability to the utmost, but rigorous proof of the restricted specificity would be impossible.

The disadvantages related to the nature of serological specificity are balanced, in part, by some advantages. Most of the antisera prepared against morphine conjugates react with glucuronide-bound morphine as well as with free morphine. The efficiency with which such sera recognize the bound drug varies from one antiserum to the other, as well as for different bleedings from the same animal. The data shown in Table 2 illustrate the range encountered in our experience. It is obvious that antisera such as 181 would facilitate the detection of total morphine while others, such as 437, would yield results more closely related to those obtained by chemical analyses of samples that had not been hydrolyzed. From a practical point of view it would indeed seem highly desirable to encourage manufacturers of diagnostic reagents to specify for each lot of antiserum its reactivity with bound drug.

Another point of importance is that antisera will bind some but not all metabolites of drugs. Since the reactivity of a given antiserum with some minor drug metabolite may be disproportionally strong, and because not all metabolites are known, the results of serological tests must be stated in terms of observed concentration of drug equivalents. Thus, in the case of morphine, the antiserum which has been calibrated against morphine will yield results that can be expressed in terms of morphine equivalents (in weight units) per unit volume of biological fluid.

In view of the considerations just stated, it appears obvious that serological tests for drugs cannot and, indeed, must not be used to prove the presence of a drug in a test specimen. Thus, they differ conceptually from the standard physico-chemical test procedures. In serological testing, it is the specimen shown to be free of detectable drug which provides the definitive answer while a specimen that appears to contain drug requires confirmation by independent test methods. Therefore, the proper use of serological testing is that of an exclusion test, much in the manner in which blood typing is used to exclude paternity and never to prove it.

If this concept is accepted, several corollaries will follow. First, it would seem advisable to use the serological tests at or near their maximal sensitivity which, under practical conditions, is about 25 ng morphine equivalents/ml undiluted urine for the radioimmunoassay and for hemagglutination-inhibition. Some laboratories concerned with the difficulty of confirming by independent tests results of serological tests which indicate the presence of less than 500 ng morphine equivalents/ml urine have elected to sacrifice sensitivity of the serological tests and have adjusted these procedures to match the sensitivity of the chromatographic assay. It is suggested that this practice should be reconsidered, especially if the concept of a valid exclusion test can be agreed upon.

Second, if future observations bear out the present impression that heroin addicts must have abstained from use of the drug for at least 3 to 4 days before the concentration of morphine in urine specimens drops below 25 ng morphine equivalents/ml, whereas morphine concentrations of greater than 500 ng/ml rarely persist for longer than 24 to 36 hr, the use of the more sensitive method recommends itself and the finding of no detectable drug at this level of sensitivity gains significance. In view of this, the cogent discussion of Goldstein and Brown[3] on the relation of test sensitivity to the required frequency of testing appears to be particularly germane.

Finally, if the principle of an exclusion test were to be applied to the problems of drug testing, the appropriate controls require discussion, especially since these would differ from standards and controls used in methods aimed at the detection and positive identification of drugs. Using the exclusion of heroin use as an example, one essential control must show that morphine (the major metabolite) can be detected under the specific conditions of the test when present in concentrations of at least 25 ng/ml. For this purpose, a standard solution of morphine in saline or in normal urine will suffice. The concentration of 25 ng/ml is suggested as suitable for the hemagglutination-inhibition test because our experience shows it to be well within the range over which most antisera yield highly reproducible results. Reasons for selecting a high level of sensitivity in the serological exclusion tests have already been discussed. The incontrovertible fact that at this level of sensitivity some specimens from users of codeine, or from individuals who have taken large doses of dextromethorphan or poppy seeds (Table 1) will not be distinguishable from specimens of heroin addicts is not relevant within the context of an exclusion test.

A second control which must be done for each specimen that is tested must ascertain that the specimen is free of activity or substances that would mask the presence of morphine. In the case of hemagglutination-inhibition this could be material that causes agglutination of the indicator cells. The precautions we use and the appropriate control are described below in the detailed description of HI test procedures. Inasmuch as the binding of morphine to glucuronide constitutes masking of a different type which varies in intensity as a function of the antiserum that is used (Table 2), it is also desirable that the relative reactivity of each antiserum with free and bound morphine be known and that antisera which react efficiently with both forms of morphine be used preferentially.

THE HEMAGGLUTINATION-INHIBITION TEST

Of the several serological test procedures that have come into use recently, hemagglutination-inhibition (HI) has been of particular concern to us. We have developed this test for the detection of morphine[4,5] and, jointly with Dr. D. Catlin, have subjected it to a limited field trial.[6] We have also adapted the test to the detection of methadone[7] and are presently working toward tests for additional drugs in which HI will be used. Procedural details have been published in the papers cited and additional information will be presented below. We shall also comment on our experience in using the test with reagents prepared either in our laboratory or in other laboratories by individuals whom we have instructed. As Catlin's data indicate,[8] HI and radioimmunoassay applied to the same specimens yielded results that were in excellent agreement.

Hemagglutination, or, more precisely, passive hemagglutination is a standard procedure of serology which allows the detection and measurement of antibodies directed against a soluble antigen which has been attached to erythrocytes either by adsorption or by chemical linkage. Such "coated" red cells serve as an indicator of the reaction between antibody and the coating antigen. In the presence of sufficient antibody, the indicator cells settle within 60 to 120 min into a film-like pattern of agglutination. In the absence of sufficient antibody, the sedimented cells form a "button" or "doughnut." The antibody content of an immune serum is generally determined in this procedure by testing serial twofold dilutions, and the highest dilution which still causes agglutination is referred to as the "titer" of the serum. Since the test is highly sensitive to antibody, titers of 10^{-4} to 10^{-7} are common for reasonably potent antisera.

A variant of this procedure, namely hemagglutination-inhibition, lends itself to the detection of soluble antigens. In the HI test, constant amounts of antiserum are incubated with a series of dilutions of the soluble antigen for a period of a few minutes before the indicator cells are added. Antibody that has been bound by the soluble antigen is, of course, no longer available for agglutination of the indicator cells and, if sufficient antibody has been bound, inhibition of hemagglutination is observed.

Since the minimal amount of soluble antigen which is required for inhibition of agglutination depends upon the amount of antibody that is used, the sensitivity of the test can be adjusted over a wide range. The working range is conveniently determined by a checkerboard titration as illustrated in Table 3. While the titer of the serum sets a limit for the minimal amount of antigen that can be detected, a limit on the maximal amount that can be measured also exists. The reason for this limitation stems from the presence in antisera of antibodies with different specificities. In the present situation, antisera prepared by immunization with carboxymethylmorphine contain some antibody that reacts with carboxymethylmorphine only and not with morphine. Since the coating antigen is carboxymethylmorphine, no reasonable amount of morphine will inhibit agglutination of such cells by this class of antibody. Fortunately, such antibody generally accounts for only a very small fraction of the total antibody and is simply diluted out. We believe that studies in progress will enable us to prepare antisera in the future which are entirely free of such antibody.

Reference to the data in Table 3 shows that this particular antiserum detected morphine in concentrations of 0.8, 3, 6 to 12 etc. ng/ml, respectively,

TABLE 3

Hemagglutination Inhibition – Checkerboard Titration

Anti-CMM serum 0.025 ml	Morphine	
	ng	ng/ml
1:100		>100
1:500		>100
1:1,000	2.5	100
1:2,000	1.2	50
1:4,000	0.6	25
1:8,000	0.15–0.3	6–12
1:16,000	0.07	3
1:32,000	0.02	0.8
1:64,000	–	–

Note: A sheep antiserum against BSA-CMM absorbed with aggregated BSA was used in this titration. The useful range extended from serum diluted 1:1,000 to 1:32,000. Beyond the last of these dilutions, agglutination no longer occurred. Agglutination by serum 1:100 could not be inhibited by 1 μg of morphine but reacted to lesser amounts of codeine and carboxymethylmorphine. See text for comments.

when used in dilutions of 1:32,000, 1:16,000, 1:8,000 etc. Since urine samples are routinely diluted 1:10 for use in the HI test, the minimal amounts that could be detected were 8 ng/ml urine when the antiserum was employed in a dilution of 1:32,000.

It has been our experience that storage of urine specimens at 4°C for several hours or preferably overnight, followed by a tenfold dilution of the clear supernatant, is sufficient preparation of the specimen for its use in the HI test. For the analysis of freshly voided specimens, we have found it adequate to chill them briefly and to subject the specimen to centrifugation in the cold. If this is omitted, agglutination of the indicator cells frequently occurs, presumably because of the precipitation of particulate materials from the urine. It is the purpose of the diluent control (mentioned below) to detect such agglutination by the specimen which might obscure the presence of morphine equivalents.

As discussed more fully in the papers cited, we consider the strength of the HI test to lie in its rapidity, simplicity, and economy. With regard to economy, it should be kept in mind that no equipment other than a clinical centrifuge is required, that the supplies are disposable glass and plastic, and that none of the reagents required are costly, exotic, or hazardous. Furthermore, since the test is a micro procedure, the absolute amounts of reagents needed are minimal. In one of several versions of the test used in the study of several thousand urine specimens, we have employed 6 cups of the standard 96-cup disposable hemagglutination tray for each urine specimen. All 6 cups are charged with 1 drop each (0.03 ml) of urine diluted 1:10. Two of the cups, the control for possible agglutination by the urine, receive 1 drop diluent and 2 other cups receive 1 drop each of antiserum diluted so that the presence of 15 to 30 ng morphine/ml urine will be revealed. The last 2 cups receive antiserum in higher concentration, so that 150 to 300 ng morphine/ml urine are required to inhibit agglutination. A list of supplies and reagents required to perform 1,000 analyses by this procedure is provided in Table 4. The amounts listed are in sufficient excess of those required to allow for losses in pipetting and for the performance of controls with known amounts of morphine.

With regard to the preparation of the reagent, a few comments appear indicated. In preparing the indicator cells, it is important to pay close attention to maintaining the proper cell concentration and to the full and complete dispersion of the rather "sticky" cells after each step and once again just before use in the test. It should also be noted that occasional lots of sheep red cells are either hyper- or hypoagglutinable, a situation with which we deal either by avoidance or by appropriate blending. Suspensions of indicator cells are stable for several days at refrigerator temperature but such stored preparations should be centrifuged and resuspended in buffer containing 1% normal rabbit serum if they are older than 24 hr. Formalinized cells, tanned and coated by the usual precedure, offer the advantage of being resistant to freezing. While they can be stored indefinitely at -20 or -70°C, it should be noted that they are more difficult to prepare. There admittedly exists an element of art in the preparation of indicator cells which, however, is readily acquired by practice and experience.

The normal rabbit serum used in the suspending medium for indicator cells and as diluent for other test reagents must be free of agglutinating action against sheep red cells and should be kept free of bacterial contamination. We screen individual sera after they have been heated at 56°C for 30 min and then prepare a pool which is divided into small portions to be stored in the freezer. We prefer to prepare the required dilutions freshly at the start of the day's work. Addition of merthiolate (1:10,000) is recommended if diluted serum is to be kept for more than 1 working day.

Our antisera are freed of antibodies to the carrier protein by preliminary absorption with heated, carbodiimide-treated bovine serum albumin. This treatment results in a tenfold dilution and such diluted serum is distributed into tubes in small amounts to be stored in the freezer. Further dilutions are made at the start of the day's work. It is our policy to start each day with a checkerboard titration in which 3 or 4 dilutions of the serum known to be the appropriate ones from earlier titrations are used against a series of dilutions of morphine (100 ng to 0.2 ng/ml). The results of this test reaffirm the proper antiserum dilutions to be used in the assays of the urine specimens.

At this time, the test is done manually. With some experience, 50 to 60 urine specimens can be tested per hr/operator. The repetitive pipettings of

TABLE 4

Reagents and Supplies for 1,000 Urine Tests

Indicator cells:

Packed sheep red cells	2.4	ml
Buffer 7.6 to prepare 3% cell suspension	80.0	ml
Tannic acid 1:1,000 in H_2O	0.8	ml
Buffer 7.6 to prepare tannic acid 1:20,000	80.0	ml
Heated bovine serum albumin-CMM (stock sol. 1 mg protein/ml)	3.2	ml
Buffer 6.5 to prepare BSA-CMM 1:100	320.0	ml
Heated normal rabbit serum	3.2	ml
Buffer 7.6 to prepare normal rabbit serum 1:100	320.0	ml

Diluent:

To dilute each of 1,000 specimens 1:10	660.0	ml
To dilute antiserum A	55.0	ml
To dilute antiserum B	55.0	ml
For control wells	55.0	ml
To prepare total diluent required		
Heated normal rabbit serum	3.4	ml
Buffer 7.6	850.0	ml

Antiserum:

To prepare 55 ml 1:1,000 (A)	0.055	ml
To prepare 55 ml 1:8,000 (B)	0.007	ml

Supplies:

Disposable tubes 10 x 75 for urine specimens	1,100
Pasteur pipettes, disposable	1,100
Hemagglutination trays, disposable	64
Calibrated dropper pipettes, 0.05 ml/drop	2
Calibrated dropper pipettes, 0.025 ml/drop	4

Note: Buffers 7.6 and 6.5, respectively, are phosphate buffers 0.075 M with respect to PO_4 and 0.075 M with respect to NaCl.

In the above scheme, it is assumed that the anti-CMM serum is such that inhibition of hemagglutination requires the presence of at least 500 ng morphine/ml urine when the serum is used in dilution 1:1,000 (A) but only 30 ng morphine/ml when the serum is used in dilution 1:8,000 (B).

diluent, the 2 dilutions of the antiserum, and of the indicator cells can be done by existing automatic pipetting equipment. While such automation would unquestionably reduce the fatigue factor, no significant saving of time would be expected. The reading of the results presents no difficulties if properly prepared reagents and acceptable technique have been employed. While we consider the technical demands of the HI procedure to be well within the capabilities of a well-trained and disciplined technician, it must be realized that the test is a highly sensitive procedure based on a delicate balance and thus requires a modicum of care in its performance.

SUMMARY

In summary, we believe that serological tests for drugs in biological fluids should properly be used at their maximal practical sensitivity and solely for the purpose of excluding the presence of the drug in question. We have discussed in some detail the application of one such test, hemagglutination-inhibition, to the detection of morphine.

REFERENCES

1. Landsteiner, K., *The Specificity of Serological Reactions,* Harvard University Press, Cambridge, Mass., 1947.

2. Beiser, S. M., Butler, V. P., Jr., and Erlanger, B. F., Haptenprotein conjugates: methodology and application, in *Textbook of Immunopathology,* Vol. I, Miescher, P. A. and Muller, H. J., Eds., Grune & Stratton, N.Y., 1968, 15.

3. Goldstein, A. and Brown, B. W., Urine testing schedules in methadone maintenance treatment of heroin addiction, *J.A.M.A.,* 214, 311, 1970.

4. Adler, F. L. and Liu, C.-T., Detection of morphine by hemagglutination-inhibition, *J. Immunol.,* 106, 1684, 1971.

5. Adler, F. L., Liu, C.-T., and Catlin, D. H., Immunological studies on heroin addiction. I. Methodology and application of a hemagglutination inhibition test for detection of morphine, *Clin. Immunol. Immunopathol.,* 1, 53, 1972.

6. Catlin, D. H., Adler, F. L., and Liu, C.-T., Immunological studies on heroin addiction. II. Applications of a sensitive hemagglutination-inhibition test for detecting morphine to diagnostic problems in chronic heroin addiction, *Clin. Immunol. Immunopathol.,* 1, 446, 1973.

7. Liu, C.-T. and Adler, F. L., Immunological studies on drug addiction. I. Antibodies reactive with methadone and their use for detection of the drug, *J. Immunol.,* 1973, in press.

8. Catlin, D. H., Urine testing: A comparison of five current methods for detecting morphine, *Am. J. Clin. Pathol.,* 111, 472, 1973.

USE OF ENZYME AND SPIN LABELING IN HOMOGENEOUS IMMUNOCHEMICAL DETECTION METHODS

R. S. Schneider

R. J. Bastiani

R. K. Leute

K. E. Rubenstein

E. F. Ullman

TABLE OF CONTENTS

INTRODUCTION

Some years ago, Spector and Parker[1] described a radioimmunoassay (RIA) for the detection of morphine and morphine-like compounds in urine and serum. This assay was described as being extremely sensitive. However, the procedure involved considerable sample manipulation and laboratory time to complete. Recent efforts by Catlin, et al.[2] have been directed toward the improvement of this technique to permit practical application to the testing of human biological fluids.

As in all radioimmunoassays, a requirement of this assay is that antigen bound to antibody must be physically separated from unbound antigen. Such a separation step is necessary because the label on the antigen is detected equally in both bound and free states. A partial solution to the problem of separation is available by the use of the hemagglutination inhibition method which has been introduced for morphine assays by Adler, et al.[3,4] Although in this method no physical separation is required, problems of nonspecific adsorption inherent in two-phase systems are still not avoided.

Immunoassay methods that employ only one phase, known as homogeneous immunoassays,[5,18] require no separation steps. One such method, FRAT® (an electron spin resonance label-immunoassay technique) has been introduced by Leute, et al.[6,7] The method employs a drug labeled with a free radical (spin label), which can be detected by an electron spin resonance spectrometer. This method has been used widely for the detection of morphine in urine. A second, related immunoassay procedure, EMIT®, which employs an enzyme in place of the spin label, has also been reported.[5,18] The term homogeneous immunoassay is used to distinguish these latter two methods from other immunoassay methods[8-12] that are "heterogeneous" and which, like radioimmunoassay, depend on the physical separation of the bound and unbound antigen.

The immunochemical methods of analyses enjoy certain advantages over chromatographic techniques. These include sensitivity, specificity, and the capability to analyze a urine specimen without sample pretreatment or extraction. Homogeneous immunoassay procedures allow this type of analysis to be performed with simplified or

This chapter was contributed by the Syva Corporation, Palo Alto California.

automated sample handling and a determination can be completed in 1 to 2 min.

Recently, immunochemical methods have been applied for the detection of abused drugs in urine. The homogeneous immunoassays for drugs of abuse are best utilized on-site in heroin treatment clinics, hospital emergency rooms, law enforcement facilities, clinical toxicology departments, medical examiners' laboratories, and in pre-employment screening or community health programs.

The purpose of this paper is to discuss in detail the principles and performance of the two homogeneous immunochemical techniques.

THE FRAT SYSTEM

FRAT General Principle

The FRAT spin immunoassay method employs the technique of spin labeling[6],[7] for the detection of antigen/antibody reactions. Nitroxide radicals are used which usually show simple three-line electron spin resonance (ESR) spectra (Figure 1) provided that the molecules can tumble freely in solution. However, if the mobility of these radicals is reduced, significant line broadening occurs, resulting in considerably decreased signal intensities (Figure 2). Such a decrease in mobility is obtained if the radical becomes bound to a large molecule, such as a protein, which tumbles relatively slowly in solution. In the spin immunoassay method nitroxide labeled haptens (drug molecules) are employed that are sufficiently small so that their ESR spectra appear as three sharp lines. However, upon binding of the labeled drug to an antibody that recognizes the drug portion of the molecule, the mobility of the radical is decreased and a broad-line spectrum is observed.

In FRAT drug abuse assays, known amounts of antibodies to the drug to be detected are mixed with an analogue of the drug that has been labeled with a nitroxide radical (spin label). The biological fluid specimen to be assayed is then added to this

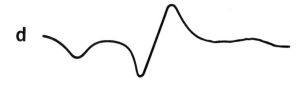

FIGURE 2.

mixture. Due to competition between the spin-labeled drug and the free drug for the limited number of antibody binding sites, some of the spin-labeled drug becomes detached from the antibody. The presence of free spin-labeled drug is signaled by the appearance of a sharp three-line ESR spectrum superimposed on the broad spectrum produced by the bound label (Figure 3).

Measurement of the intensity of either the high or low field peaks provides a direct measure for the drug concentration. A schematic representation of the process is shown in Figure 4.

Antisera to the drugs to be assayed were obtained by injection of protein conjugates of the drugs into goats or sheep. The γ-globulin fractions of the serum samples were separated by ammonium sulfate precipitation. Association constants of the antibodies with the free drug were usually in the range of 10^6 to 10^8.

The 2,2,5,5-tetramethyl-1-pyrrolidinyloxyl group was employed as the nitroxide radical to tag the drug molecule. Usually the same site on the drug was used for attachment to both the spin label and the protein carrier. This resulted in good recognition of the spin-labeled drugs by the antibodies, and, in fact, affinities of the antibodies for the spin labels were often greater than for the free drugs.

Assay Method

In addition to the FRAT spectrometer which is an electron spin resonance instrument, certain ancillary supplies are needed to facilitate the analysis. These include syringes, calibrated microcapillaries, and disposable beakers.

Performing a FRAT drug abuse assay involves drawing 50 microliters of an untreated urine sample into a calibrated capillary pipette. The sample is then deposited in a small plastic beaker containing 5 μl of an oxidizing agent (dichromate). A 20-μl aliquot of the urine-dichromate mixture is then transferred with the same capillary to a second beaker containing 10 μl of previously mixed antibody and spin-labeled drug. This com-

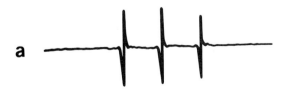

FIGURE 1.

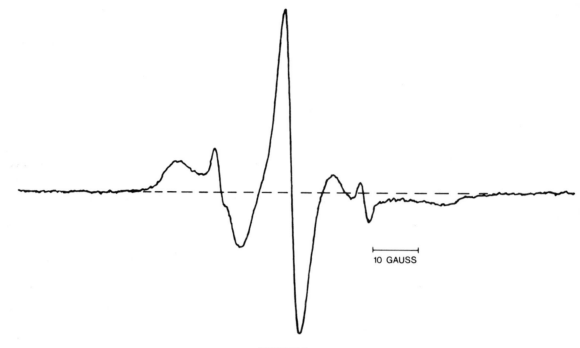

FIGURE 3.

bined solution is drawn into the capillary, the tip is sealed with putty, and the solution allowed to equilibrate for 15 to 30 min. After this interval, the capillary is placed in the FRAT spectrometer. The instrument traces the reading within 30 sec. Up to 600 assays can be performed on a FRAT instrument in an 8-hr day.

The concentration of drug in the urine is determined by comparison with urine-based calibrators containing known concentrations of drug. For mass screening when it is only necessary to establish if a minimum predetermined concentration of the drug is present, peak heights of biological specimens can be compared with the peak height produced by a suitable calibrator.

Samples that give signals below this cutoff value are taken to be negative; samples giving higher signals are called positive.

A quantitative result can be obtained by comparison with the signal intensity of known standards. A standard curve (Figure 5) is prepared by plotting the calibrator concentrations against the corresponding peak heights.

FRAT calibrators are prepared from standard solutions of drugs in drug free human urine. For stability purposes, the calibrators are supplied as lyophilized powders which are reconstituted with distilled water before use. Upon reconstitution the calibrators contain the following concentration of drugs ($\mu g/ml$).

Calibrator	Negative	Low	Medium	High
Morphine	0	0.5	5.0	50
Methadone	0	0.5	5.0	50
Amphetamine	0	1.0	5.0	50
Secobarbital	0	1.0	5.0	50
Benzoyl ecgonine (cocaine metabolite)	0	1.0	5.0	50

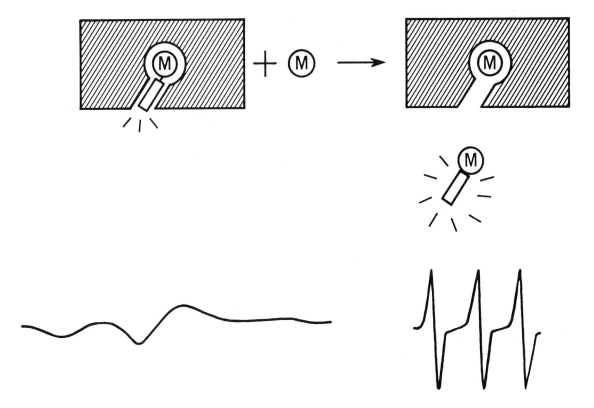

FIGURE 4.

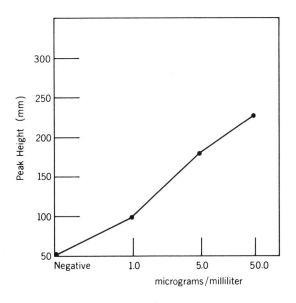

FIGURE 5.

Once reconstituted, the solutions are stable for 2 weeks if maintained at 4°C when not in use.

The FRAT assays are designed with a dynamic range covering two orders of magnitude (0.5 to 50 μg/ml). Most accurate quantitation is achieved in the first decade (0.5 to 5.0 μg/ml). Above this level, assay response is somewhat less sensitive. In order to achieve accurate quantitation on samples of greater than 5.0 μg/ml concentrations, these high specimens should be quantitatively diluted with a negative urine calibrator and reassayed.

FRAT Assays

The five FRAT assays for the detection of abuse drugs and their sensitivities to related drugs are listed in Table 1.

The detection level for each assay was determined from histograms such as those shown in Appendix 1. The histograms give the variation in FRAT readings of selected negative urine specimens together with data for the same 100 urines to which known drugs of various concentrations were added ("spiked urines").

TABLE 1

FRAT Drug Abuse Assays

FRAT assay	Drugs detected	Cutoff level* (μg/ml)	Corresponding detection level μg/ml
Opiates	Codeine		0.1
	Morphine	0.25	0.5
	Morphine glucuronide		1.5
	Heroin		1.5
Methadone	Methadone	0.25	0.50
	Alpha-acetylmethadol		0.50
Barbiturate	Secobarbital	1.0	2.0
	Phenobarbital		2.8
	Pentobarbital		4.5
	Amobarbital		6.8
	Butabarbital		13.0
Amphetamine	Amphetamine	1.0	3.0
	Methamphetamine		4.4
Cocaine Metabolite	Benzoylecgonine	0.5	1.0
	Ecgonine		12.0

*The cutoff level is the concentration of drug in a calibrator solution which will give a minimum reading below which samples will be deemed negative. This level is set so that greater than 95% of the samples containing drug at the detection level will be identified as positive.

The histograms shown are for urines spiked at the suggested detection levels. These levels were established by the requirement that there be some FRAT reading given by the histogram which falls below 95% of the readings of the spiked samples and above 95% of the readings of the negative samples.

The most effective use of the FRAT data requires the selection of a specific minimum peak height that will denote the presence of a drug in the specimen. Samples which give signals greater than this cutoff can then be designated as positives. The most satisfactory cutoff will usually be that signal which permits correct identification of >95% of all positives and of all negatives. However, some laboratories find it convenient to use higher cutoffs to avoid false-positive readings despite the concomitant decreased probability of detection of very low drug concentrations.

To illustrate the importance of this point, the histogram for the FRAT Methadone Assay is reproduced in Figure 6. Examination of this histogram shows that the selection of 96 mm as the cutoff signal height should produce about 2% false-positive responses as a result of high background samples. However, virtually all the samples which contain 0.5 μg/ml of methadone would be detected.

If this incidence of false-positive responses is undesirable, a sufficiently high cutoff can be chosen to avoid this problem. Thus, a cutoff signal height of 127 mm (center of the 0.5 μg/ml distribution) would still permit detection of 50% of all samples containing 0.5 μg/ml of methadone and, of course, very much higher percentages of all samples with greater than 0.5 μg/ml methadone.

Thus, histograms allow a laboratory to select a cutoff point which best fulfills its requirements. If ultimate sensitivity is required, the histogram can be used to determine the false-positive rate which can be expected. If no false-positive determinations can be tolerated, an appropriately higher cutoff can be selected with knowledge concerning the false-negative rates that will result.

It should be apparent that the reproducibility of *all* analytical methods including TLC, GLC, UV, fluorometry, and other immunoassays show urine-to-urine variations caused by differences in urine composition. Thus, similar studies are required for each of these procedures in order to select valid detection criteria.

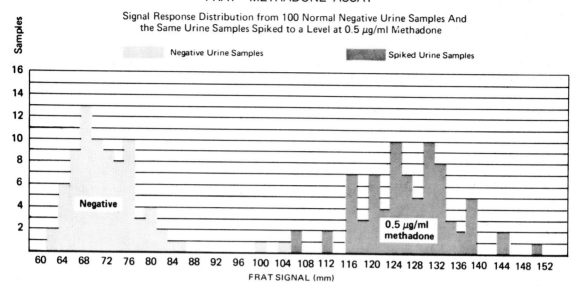

FRAT® METHADONE ASSAY

Signal Response Distribution from 100 Normal Negative Urine Samples And
the Same Urine Samples Spiked to a Level at 0.5 µg/ml Methadone

FIGURE 6.

Assay Specificity

Antibodies employed in immunochemical assays for small molecules are usually produced by injection of animals with protein conjugates of an analogue of the specific molecule toward which antibodies are desired. The natural immune defense mechanism of the animals leads to the formation of the required antibodies which may be isolated from the serum.

Despite the highly selective binding by antibodies, immunochemical assays are seldom monospecific. At sufficiently high concentrations, compounds chemically related to the compound of interest will frequently bind to the antibodies. The cross-reactivities of the FRAT assays, both desirable and undesirable, are listed in Appendix 2.

Very frequently the immune response of an animal can be at least partially controlled to yield antisera of desired specificity. In the case of the FRAT Opiate Assay, the specificity of the antibody is designed to detect not only morphine but also morphine glucuronide, which is the primary urinary excretion product of heroin. The significance of detecting both free and conjugated morphine was established in studies by Way and Adler[13] in which they demonstrated that more than 80% of the total morphine excreted is in the conjugated form. Thus, it is essential that a morphine analysis procedure be capable of responding to the major metabolic product in order

to detect samples containing low opiate concentrations.

Likewise, the FRAT Barbiturate Assay is designed to detect the more common barbiturates as a class rather than identify an individual barbiturate. This broad specificity was incorporated into the assay since many members of the class are abused.

The FRAT Amphetamine Assay also detects amphetamine analogues as a class, and is therefore equally sensitive to methamphetamine and to the parent compound. Other phenylethylamines such as mephentermine and phentermine can also be detected, but only at higher concentrations. Cross-reactivity to phenylpropanolamine and ephedrine is also observed at high concentrations. Since these latter two compounds are found in some cold remedies and bronchodilators, all FRAT amphetamine-positive specimens should be confirmed by an alternate nonimmunochemical methodology.

In contrast, The Methadone and Cocaine Metabolite Assays are extremely selective in the compounds to which the assay will respond since, in these cases, it is most desirable to detect only one member of the class.

Clinical Results

The introduction of the FRAT Cocaine Metabolite Assay was a significant advancement for the detection of cocaine abuse. Early techniques were successful only in detecting very recent gross abuse of cocaine, and were unable to detect this drug beyond 12 to 24 hr after its use. Low doses were often not detected.[17] Since this FRAT assay has been available for only a short time, a detailed discussion of the clinical performance is appropriate. Performance of the remaining four FRAT assays, particularly opiates, has been previously discussed.[19,20]

The FRAT system allows detection of the primary urinary cocaine excretion product, benzoyl ecgonine, at a cutoff level of 1 μg/ml. Urine specimens from patients given cocaine were analyzed by the FRAT Cocaine Metabolite Assay. These samples were found to contain detectable amounts of benzoyl ecgonine 24 to 48 hr after the drug ingestion.

The results for five patients in the study are shown in Figure 7. The initial dose of cocaine was not controlled, and thus might have differed for each subject shown.

A reliability study of this assay was conducted by supplying sets of twenty benzoylecgonine-spiked urine samples to various cooperating laboratories for FRAT analysis. These samples contained a variety of drugs at several concentrations. All of the samples containing benzoylecgonine were between 2.0 and 10 μg/ml. The analyst was instructed to analyze each unknown for benzoyl ecgonine with the FRAT Cocaine Metabolite Assay.

Employing a 1.0-μg/ml cutoff, all 36 urines spiked above this level were correctly reported as positive by all of the participating laboratories.

The accuracy of the FRAT quantitation achieved with these same sets of spiked urines is summarized in Table 2.

The specificity of the Cocaine Metabolite Assay is such that only benzoyl ecgonine and, to a lesser degree, ecgonine are detected (see Appendix 2). To verify that no other common drugs or their metabolite interfere with the assay, a series of 300 urine samples from hospital patients were analyzed

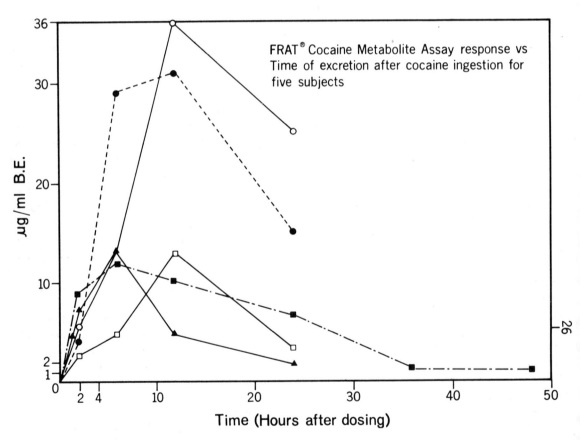

FRAT® Cocaine Metabolite Assay response vs Time of excretion after cocaine ingestion for five subjects

FIGURE 7.

TABLE 2

FRAT Cocaine Metabolite Assay Quantitative Comparison of Spiked Sample

	Benzoyl ecgonine concentration μg/ml			
Laboratory	2.0*	5.0*	10.0	Average deviation from mean
San Francisco Bay area	1.8	4.6	8.0	0.13
Pacific Northwest	1.75	3.9	12.0	1.44
Los Angeles area	2.0	3.85	6.0	0.84
Syva	1.73	4.5	6.0	0.79
Mean	1.8	4.2	8.0	
Standard deviation	0.12	0.39	2.8	

*Several samples were spiked at this level. For the purpose of this tabulation, the results from all samples that contained equivalent concentrations were averaged.

with the Cocaine Metabolite Assay. These specimens contained from 1 to 10 drugs each. Due to the controlled hospital environment, it was possible to ascertain that none of these samples contained cocaine. All analyses were negative, i.e., their assay response for benzoyl ecgonine was less than 1.0 μg/ml.

The importance of a zero false-positive rate is amplified by the lack of nonimmunological confirmatory methods of equal sensitivity to the FRAT assay. Existing TLC or GLC procedures[21] have sensitivities that are not equivalent to the immunochemical method.

THE EMIT SYSTEM

Introduction

In the previous section, the spin immunoassay or FRAT technique was described in detail. The use of a drug labeled with a free radical (spin label) is but one example of the general concept of homogeneous immunoassays. Another example of a related immunoassay procedure employs an enzyme in place of a free radical as a label. This technique, identified commercially as the EMIT System, is illustrated in Figure 8. In the method used for drug abuse detection a drug is labeled

with the enzyme lysozyme. Lysozyme catalyzes the lysis of bacteria by effecting the breakdown of the bacterial cell walls. When the enzyme-labeled drug is complexed with sheep or rabbit antibody to the drug, the enzyme is rendered inactive. The exact mechanism for the enzyme inactivation is not known but it is postulated to arise by steric exclusion of the enzyme substrate from the enzyme active site. In the presence of free drug or related compounds, the lysozyme drug conjugate and free drug compete for antibody binding sites. Thus, the presence of the free drug causes some of the lysozyme drug conjugate to remain uncomplexed and enzymatically active. The level of enzyme activity is directly related to the concentration of free drug introduced.

This technique has the potential for very great sensitivity because of the possibility for chemical amplification. Thus, one molecular event, the release of a molecule of lysozyme drug conjugate, can cause the conversion of many molecules of substrate to product. The ultimate sensitivity of the method is, of course, dependent upon the choice of enzyme and the method employed for determination of the reaction rate. Since extremely high sensitivity ($<$ 300 ng/ml) is not required for detection of many drugs of abuse, the present EMIT assay has been tailored to take advantage of some of the other unique advantages of this methodology. These include simplicity of sample handling and immediacy of results made possible by the avoidance of a separation step, use of standard spectrophotometers available in many clinical laboratories, ease of automation, and avoidance of unstable radioactive reagents. In a semiautomated commercial form of the assay, determination of a single urine sample can be completed within a few minutes once a standard curve has been prepared.

We propose the term, homogeneous enzyme immunoassay,[5] to distinguish the method from other enzyme immunoassay methods that are "heterogeneous" and which, like radioimmunoassay, depend on the physical separation of the bound and unbound antigen.

Instrumentation

The same instrumentation can be used to perform all of the EMIT drug assays.

1. **Spectrophotometer** — The assay is performed on a spectrophotometer equipped with a

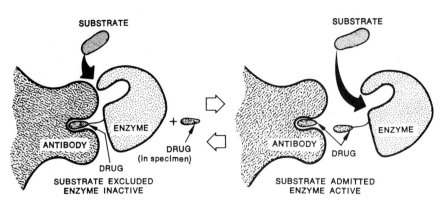

SUBSTRATE EXCLUDED
ENZYME INACTIVE

SUBSTRATE ADMITTED
ENZYME ACTIVE

FIGURE 8.

37°C thermally regulated micro flow cell. A suitable instrument is the Gilford 300-N Spectrometer equipped with Model 3017 Thermo Cuvette.

2. **Printer** — An EMIT automatic printer (Model 5B069) supplied by Syva Company is employed. The instrument permits the operator to record a sample number and obtain a printed record of the result including the initial and final absorbances and the change in absorbance. In addition, the instrument controls the timing of the assay.

3. **Diluter/pipette** — It is convenient to use an automatic diluter/pipette capable of sampling 50 µl of a urine sample and delivering the sample plus 250 µl of buffer.

Reagents

Three EMIT reagents are required for each assay. These reagents are (1) an antibody prepared against a particular drug or drug metabolite, (2) a lysozyme drug conjugate, and (3) the enzyme substrate. The antibodies are prepared in rabbits and sheep according to standard procedures. The preparation of the lysozyme drug conjugates is similar to the preparation of the antigen. The most useful conjugates were shown to have 4 to 5 antigens per lysozyme by use of radio-labeled material. These reagents are stable for a least 1 year if stored at 4°C. The enzyme substrate, *Micrococcus luteus,* is a nonpathogenic bacterium which is supplied as a lyophilized powder. After reconstitution, the suspension is usable for seven days if kept at 4°C when not in use.

Calibrators

Normal human urine was collected from healthy drug-free adults. After showing that each sample did not give an appreciably different result from buffer in the EMIT assay for opiates, barbiturates, methadone, benzoyl ecgonine, and amphetamine, the samples were pooled and filtered. The urine calibrators were prepared from a combination of the drugs for which EMIT assays are available. Stock solution containing 50 µg/ml of each drug in pooled human urine was prepared and diluted with different amounts of pooled normal urine to give the low, medium, and high calibrator concentrations shown in Figure 9. The calibrators are lyophilized. Once reconstituted with distilled water, the calibrators may be retained up to 14 days if kept at 4°C when not is use.

The set of urine calibrators may be used to prepare a standard curve for each of the five assays. The four-calibrator concentrations are sufficient to prepare a standard curve suitable for semiquantitative assignment of drug concentration in an unknown sample. If more accuracy is required, additional concentrations of drug should be included in the preparation of the standard curve. No cross-reactivity was found between these drug classes.

Test Procedure

Since all EMIT assays are performed in exactly the same manner, the exact assay procedure will be described in detail for only one assay.

In the performance of the EMIT opiate assay (Figure 10) a urine sample (50 µl) (no hydrolysis or extraction is required) is added to 200 µl of the enzyme substrate by means of the diluter (Step 1). Next, using the same technique, 50 µl of morphine antibody (Reagent A) is added followed by a 50 µl sample of the enzyme-labeled morphine (Reagent

EMIT Calibrators when reconstituted contain the following concentrations of drugs (μg/ml):

	Neg.	Low	Med.	High
Morphine	0.0	0.5	5.0	50.0
Methadone	0.0	0.5	5.0	50.0
Amphetamine	0.0	1.0	5.0	50.0
Secobarbital	0.0	1.0	5.0	50.0
Benzoyl Ecgonine (Cocaine metabolite)	0.0	1.0	5.0	50.0

FIGURE 9.

B). The reaction mixture (total volume 1.1 ml) is then aspirated into the spectrophotometer which automatically activates the EMIT printer.

After a 7-sec delay for thermal equilibration, the initial absorbance is printed. Forty seconds later a second absorbance is measured and printed followed by a print out of the difference between these values (ΔOD or EMIT Units). During the 47-sec measurement period all the reagents for the next sample, except the enzyme reagent, may be mixed. The amount of drug in the sample can be determined by reference to a standard curve (Figure 11) prepared by employing the calibrators.

Since there is a small chance that a positive result is due to the presence of the lysozyme in the urine, under certain circumstances it may be desirable to run a blank. This is done by employing precisely the same procedure with the exception that buffer is used in place of the enzyme and antibody reagents. The correct test result is obtained by subtracting the blank from the experimental value. Only one blank determination is required per sample because the same value can be used for all assays.

Opiate Assay[18]
General Discussion

The antibodies employed in the assay were specifically selected[6,7,15] to permit the detection of both morphine and morphine glucuronide, the major metabolites of heroin. The detection of morphine glucuronide is a significant factor. Studies by Way and Adler[13] have shown that more than 80% of the excreted morphine in urine is in the form of morphine glucuronide. Since in certain individuals practically no free morphine is found, it is essential that a procedure for detection of heroin use be capable of responding to this major metabolic product.

The assay also detects other opiates (see Table 3), including heroin, codeine, somewhat higher concentrations of the narcotic antagonist nalorphine, and the analgesic meperidine. False-positives due to cross-reactivity with non-opiate substances following their normal therapeutic use

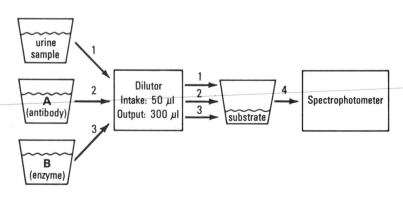

FIGURE 10.

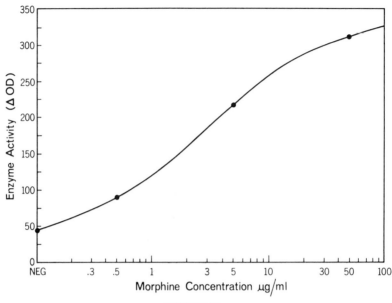

FIGURE 11.

have seldom been observed. Very high concentrations of phenothiozines e.g., chlorpromazine) and abuse concentrations of dextromethorphan are the only documented exceptions, although studies of these drugs have failed to give false-positive results when therapeutic dosages were used.

The data given in Table 3 are based on concentrations of the drugs added to normal urine. Because of the undesirability of cross-reactivity to dextromethorphan and chlorpromazine in an opiate assay, the reactivity of *metabolized* samples

of these two drugs was determined in two separate studies.

In the first study, 50 urine specimens from volunteers taking the recommended daily dosage of cough medicine (i.e., Robitussin®, Pertussin®, or Vicks 44®) were collected before medication and at 4-hr intervals for 24 hr. The results of the analysis of these samples are listed in Table 4. The assay response to the metabolized dextromethorphan is expressed in terms of the equivalent morphine concentration.

Only three samples were found to give an assay response ≥ 0.3 μg/ml. No determinations were found to produce the 0.5 μg/ml assay response necessary to give a false positive result. It is thus concluded that recommended doses of cough medications containing dextromethorphan do not interfere with the assay.

In the second study, 20 urine specimens were

TABLE 3

Relative Opiate Assay Sensitivity to Some Common Drugs

Drug	Typical concentrations in aqueous solution giving an EMIT reading equivalent to 0.5 μg/ml morphine
Codeine	0.35 μg/ml
Morphine	0.5 μg/ml
Nalorphine	5.5 μg/ml
Heroin	5.5 μg/ml
Meperidine	35.0 μg/ml
Dextromethorphan	150.0 μg/ml
Diphenoxylate	>80.0 μg/ml
Chlorpromazine	86.0 μg/ml
Naloxone	120.0 μg/ml
Methadone	500.0 μg/ml
Dextropropoxyphene	>700.0 μg/ml
Alpha-acetylmethadol	>1,000.0 μg/ml

TABLE 4

Metabolized Dextromethorphan Cross-reactivity with the EMIT Opiate Assay

Number of samples	Morphine equivalent conc. (μg/ml)
47	<0.3
2	0.3
1	0.4

TABLE 5

Equivalent Reactivity of Metabolized Chlorpromazine Samples on the EMIT Opiate Assay

Number of samples	Morphine equivalent conc. (μg/ml)
16	<0.3
3	0.31
1	0.33

obtained from hospital patients who were on prescribed doses of chlorpromazine. The doses ranged from 100 to 600 mg/day and the methods of administration included oral tablet, Spansule®, liquid or intramuscular injection. The assay response to the metabolized chlorpromazine is expressed in terms of the equivalent morphine concentration (Table 5).

No analysis resulted in an equivalent morphine concentration higher than 0.33 μg/ml, which is significantly lower than our recommended 0.5 μg/ml positive cutoff. It thus appears that chlorpromazine and/or its metabolites do not interfere with the assay at these therapeutic doses.

Detection Level and Interpretation of Data for Opiate Assay

To employ most effectively the homogeneous enzyme immunoassay for morphine, it is necessary to select a specific minimum reading that will signal the presence of morphin in the sample. Samples that give readings above this cutoff value will be identified as positive. All others will be considered negative. Selection of a low cutoff value will increase the probability of identifying positive samples, but will increase the risk of obtaining false-positives.

Preparation of the histogram given in Figure 12 permitted selection of an appropriate cutoff value. Variations in the assay response from 100 randomly selected normal urines are illustrated on the left side of the histogram and variations in the response from the same urines spiked with 0.5 μg/ml of morphine are illustrated on the right side. The data show that samples containing 0.5 μg/ml of morphine will assay for 0.5 ± 0.20 μg/ml, and negative samples will assay below 0.25 μg/ml greater than 95% of the time. In this study, lysozyme blanks were subtracted only from readings in excess of 0.3 μg/ml.

Based on this and other histograms, we have

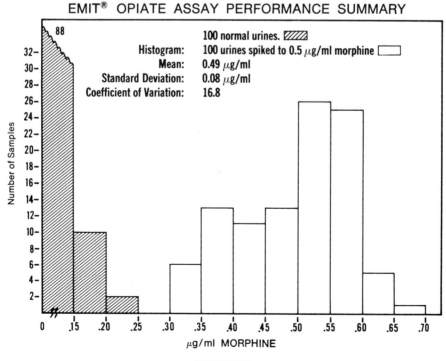

FIGURE 12.

found it convenient to use the low-calibrator reading (0.5 μg/ml of morphine) as the cutoff. Although the data show that a lower cutoff is acceptable, use of the 0.5-μg/ml cutoff introduces only about 1% false-positives due to endogenous lysozyme, a sufficiently low incidence of false-positives so that lysozyme blanks need not be run for many applications. Using the 0.5 μg/ml cutoff greater than 95% of samples containing 0.7 μg/ml of morphine are detected. A 0.3 μg/ml cutoff is required to detect with 95% confidence samples containing 0.5 μg/ml morphine.

Opiate Assay Reliability
Precision

The precision of the opiate enzyme immunoassay was shown by spiking two samples of pooled normal urine with 0.5 and 3.0 μg/ml morphine, respectively. Each sample was then analyzed repetitively by a single operator and the mean, standard deviation, and coefficient of variation were calculated at both concentrations. The results indicate the assay to have a coefficient of variation of 5.0 and 9.4% at 0.5 and 3.0 μg/ml morphine, respectively.

In another study, morphine was added to normal human urine to produce solutions from 0.7 to 5.0 μg/ml. These solutions plus a number of drug-free urines were then assayed by six different technicians in laboratories in different locations to determine the precision of the opiate enzyme immunoassay as a function of variables introduced by the operators and in different laboratory conditions. Each of the technicians correctly identified all of the drug containing samples. In addition, satisfactory quantitative precision between those participating in the study was obtained (Table 6). The average error between the spiked value and the mean assay result was 0.13 μg/ml.

Methadone Assay
General Discussion

The antibodies employed in this assay were specifically designed to permit the detection of unmetabolized methadone. Methadone when used in the treatment of heroin addiction must be administered daily and is excreted in urine both as the unmetabolized drug and one major metabolite (2-ethylidene-1,5-dimethyl-3,3-diphenyl-pyrrolidine).[16] If methadone administration is interrupted, the level of unmetabolized drug decreases rapidly, while a significant level of metabolite often persists for many days. The EMIT methadone assay was designed to detect methadone and not its major metabolite. By use of this assay, a drug treatment program has a technique available to detect when a patient volun-

TABLE 6

Effect of Operator Experience and Environment on EMIT® Opiate Assay Results *

| Operator experience (days) | Laboratory | Morphine concentration (μg/ml) | | | | | | | Average deviation from mean |
		0.7	1.0	1.5	2.0	2.5	4.0	5.0	
4	Syva	0.60	0.84	1.4	1.8	2.3	3.3	3.5	0.07
7	A	0.83	0.78	1.3	1.6	2.2	3.1	3.7	0.14
7	B	0.62	0.82	1.4	2.5	2.4	3.3	3.7	0.12
14	C	0.65	0.88	1.3	1.8	2.2	3.3	3.9	0.07
30	D	0.51	0.81	1.4	1.75	2.3	3.3	4.0	0.09
60	Syva	0.63	0.95	1.5	2.0	2.3	3.6	3.7	0.09
	Mean	0.64	0.85	1.38	1.91	2.28	3.32	3.75	
	Standard deviation	0.11	0.06	0.08	0.29	0.07	0.16	0.18	

*Each number represents an average of the values obtained from one to four different urine samples.

tarily interrupts his methadone therapy and abstains from its use.

The assay also detects other substances (see Table 7) including alpha-acetylmethadol and somewhat higher concentrations of promethazine and chlorpromazine (other phenothiazines were not tested). False positives, due to cross-reactivity with nonmethadone substances, have seldom been observed. The data in Table 7 are based on spiked concentrations of the drugs in water.

Detection Level and Interpretation of Data for Methadone Assay

The selection of a specific minimum reading that will signal the presence of methadone in a sample is most effectively illustrated by the preparation of the histogram shown in Figure 13. Based on this histogram, it is convenient to use the low-calibrator reading (0.5 μg/ml of methadone) as the cutoff. Although the data show that a lower cutoff is acceptable, use of the 0.5 μg/ml cutoff introduces only about 1% false-positives due to endogenous lysozyme. Using this cutoff, greater than 95% of the samples containing 0.7 μg/ml of methadone are detected. In order to detect 0.5

TABLE 7

Drug	Typical concentrations in aqueous solution giving an EMIT reading equivalent to 0.5 μg/ml methadone
Methadone	0.5 μg/ml
Alpha-acetylmethadol	3.0 μg/ml
Promethazine	>1,000.0 μg/ml
Chlorpromazine	150.0 μg/ml
Dextromethorphan	360.0 μg/ml
Meperidine	>300.0 μg/ml
Morphine	>1,000.0 μg/ml
Codeine	>1,000.0 μg/ml
Dextropropoxyphene	>500.0 μg/ml
Naloxone	>600.0 μg/ml
Heroin	>1,000.0 μg/ml

μg/ml of methadone at the same level of confidence, a cutoff of 0.3 μg/ml is recommended.

Performance Summary

The precision of the methadone enzyme immunoassay was shown by spiking two normal urine pools with 0.7 and 5.0 μg/ml methadone, respectively. The samples were then analyzed repetitively by a single operator to determine the

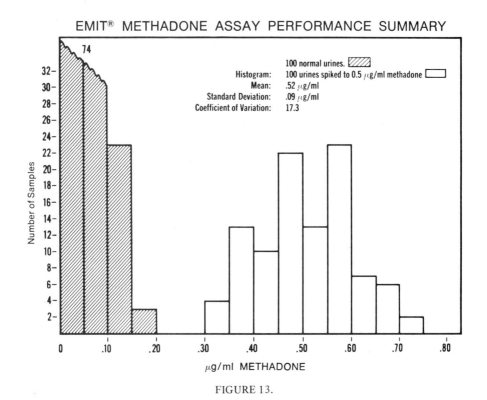

FIGURE 13.

coefficient of variation. The results indicate the assay to have a coefficient of variation of 3.8% at both the 0.7 and 5.0 μg/ml methadone levels.

A series of drug-free and methadone-spiked urines was assayed by six different technicians in laboratories in different locations to determine the precision of the methadone enzyme immunoassay as a function of variables introduced by the operators and the different laboratory conditions. Each of the technicians correctly identified all of the drug containing samples and, in addition, satisfactory quantitative precision between those participating in the study was obtained. (See Table 8)

Barbiturate Assay

General Discussion

The EMIT barbiturate assay has been designed to permit the detection of many of the common barbiturates including secobarbital, amobarbital, phenobarbital, butabarbital, and pentobarbital. However, on the basis of this assay, a positive result does not permit the determination of which of these compounds is actually present in the sample. The assay detects other barbiturates with diminished sensitivity as shown in Table 9. False-positives due to cross-reactivity with nonbarbiturate substances has not been observed.

TABLE 9

Relative Barbiturate Assay Sensitivity to Some Common Drugs

Drug	Typical concentrations in aqueous solution giving an EMIT reading equivalent to 2.0 μg/ml secobarbital
Mephobarbital	1.3 μg/ml
Pentobarbital	1.3 μg/ml
Secobarbital	2.0 μg/ml
Amobarbital	0.5 μg/ml
Phenobarbital	1.0 μg/ml
Thiopental	4.2 μg/ml
Talbutal	8.4 μg/ml
Butabarbital	2.0 μg/ml
Aprobarbital	90.0 μg/ml
Glutethimide	>100.0 μg/ml
Thiamylal	>100.0 μg/ml
Metharbital	>100.0 μg/ml
Barbital	>100.0 μg/ml
Probarbital	>100.0 μg/ml
Dilantin[®]	>100.0 μg/ml

Detection Level and Interpretation of Data for Barbiturate Assay

To employ most effectively the EMIT assay for barbiturates, it is necessary to select a specific minimum reading that will signal the presence of a barbiturate in the sample. Samples that give readings above this cutoff value will be identified

TABLE 8

Effect of Operator Experience and Environment on EMIT-Methadone Assay Results.*

Operator experience (days)	Laboratory	Methadone concentration (μg/ml)							Average deviation from mean
		0.7	1.0	1.5	2.0	3.0	4.0	6.0	
4	Syva	0.8	1.05	1.5	2.1	2.8	4.15	3.7	0.52
7	West Coast	0.9	1.38	1.7	2.55	3.5	4.1	5.6	0.23
7	West Coast	0.8	1.14	2.5	2.50	4.6	4.65	8.0	0.66
14	West Coast	0.9	1.43	2.2	2.9	4.2	4.63	8.0	0.71
30	East Coast	–	0.67	1.2	1.2	2.2	2.35	6.3	0.79
60	Syva	0.76	1.02	1.1	1.9	2.8	3.6	5.8	0.33
Mean		0.83	1.11	1.7	2.2	3.35	3.92	6.2	
Standard deviation		0.06	0.34	0.55	0.65	0.92	1.00	1.6	

*One to four different urine samples were analyzed at each concentration by each operator. Average results are presented for all equal concentration samples.

as positive. All others will be considered negative.

Preparation of the histogram given in Figure 14 permits the selection of an appropriate cutoff value. Variations in the assay response from 100 randomly selected normal urines are illustrated on the left side of the histogram and variation in the response from the same urine spiked with 2.0 μg/ml secobarbital are illustrated on the right side. The data show that samples containing 2.0 μg/ml secobarbital will assay for 2.0 ± 1.4 μg/ml, and negative samples will assay below 0.7 μg/ml greater than 95% of the time. Based on this histogram, we recommend the use of the low-calibrator reading (1.0 μg/ml secobarbital) as the cutoff. Using this cutoff, greater than 90% of the samples containing 1.0 μg/ml of secobarbital will be detected.

Performance Summary

The precision of the barbiturate enzyme immunoassay was shown by spiking two samples of pooled normal urine with 3.0 and 10.0 μg/ml secobarbital, respectively. Each sample was then analyzed repetitively by a single operator to determine the coefficient of variation of the assay. The results indicate the assay to have coefficients of variation of 9.13 and 4.8 at secobarbital

concentrations of 3.0 and 10.0 μg/ml, respectively.

A series of drug-free and secobarbital-spiked urines was assayed by four different technicians in laboratories in different locations to determine the precision of the barbiturate enzyme immunoassay as a function of laboratory variables. Each of the technicians correctly identified all of the drug containing samples and, in addition, satisfactory quantitative precision between those participating in the study was obtained (see Table 10).

General Summary of EMIT Amphetamine and Benzoyl Ecgonine (Cocaine Metabolite) Assay

Amphetamine Assay

The EMIT Amphetamine Assay has been designed principally to detect amphetamine and methamphetamine in an untreated urine sample. Certain other amphetamine-like compounds can also be detected (see Table 11).

Since high concentrations of certain other phenethylamines are occasionally detected, the assay is best used as a screening procedure and not as an absolute test for amphetamine. Syva provides an EMIT Amphetamine Confirmation reagent which when added to urine destroys many of the most commonly used phenethylamines such as

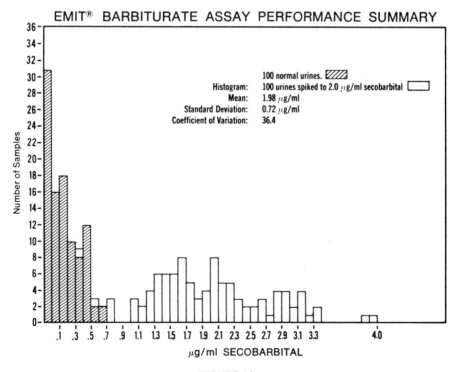

FIGURE 14.

TABLE 10

Effect of Operator Experience and Environment on EMIT Barbiturate Assay Results.*

Operator experience (days)	Laboratory	Barbiturate concentration (μg/ml)**					Average deviation from mean
		1.5	2.0	3.0	4.0	7.0	
7	West Coast	0.90	0.96	2.2	2.6	4.0	0.62
7	West Coast	0.91	1.35	2.5	2.6	5.5	0.18
30	East Coast	1.25	2.2	4.0	–	9.0	1.05
60	Syva	1.3	1.4	2.3	2.6	5.0	0.32
Mean		1.09	1.47	2.75	2.6	5.88	
Standard deviation		0.21	0.52	0.84	0.0	2.17	

*One to four different urine samples were analyzed at each concentration by each operator. Average results are presented for all equal concentration samples.

**Spiked concentration.

ephedrine and phenylpropranolamine, but does not alter amphetamine or methamphetamine. If confirmation of a positive result is required, this reagent is added to the urine sample as well as to the calibrator, and the samples are reassayed. It will usually be convenient to run the confirmatory test only on samples which have previously been found to be positive by the EMIT Amphetamine Assay.

TABLE 11

Detectability Limits

Drug	Typical concentrations in aqueous solution giving an EMIT reading equivalent to 3.0 μg/ml amphetamine
Mephentermine	1.7 μg/ml
Phentermine	1.7 μg/ml
Methamphetamine	2.0 μg/ml
Amphetamine	3.0 μg/ml
Phenmetrazine	8.3 μg/ml
Cyclopentamine	9.6 μg/ml
Benzphetamine	12.5 μg/ml
Phenylpropanolamine	16.0 μg/ml
Ephedrine	22.0 μg/ml
Nylidrin	30.0 μg/ml
Methoxyphenamine	75.0 μg/ml
Isoxsuprine	100.0 μg/ml
Methylphenidate	>1,000.0 μg/ml

Preparation of the histogram shown in Figure 15 from 100 normal urines and 100 urines spiked with 3.0 μg/ml amphetamine permits the selection of an appropriate cutoff vlaue. The data show that samples containing 3.0 μg/ml amphetamine will assay for 3.0 ± 1.5 μg/ml, and negative samples will assay below 1.0 μg/ml greater than 95% of the time.

Performance Summary: Amphetamine Assay

The precision of the amphetamine enzyme immunoassay was shown by the addition of 1.0 and 10.0 μg/ml of amphetamine to two urine pools. Each was analyzed repetitively by a single operator to determine coefficients of variation of 10.5 and 9.7 for the 1.0 and 10.0 μg/ml samples, respectively.

A series of drug-free and amphetamine-spiked urines was assayed by five different technicians in laboratories in different geographic locations to determine the precision of the amphetamine assay as a function of variables introduced by the operators and the different laboratory conditions. Each of the technicians correctly identified the drug containing samples and, in addition, satisfactory quantitative precision between those participating in the study was obtained (see Table 12).

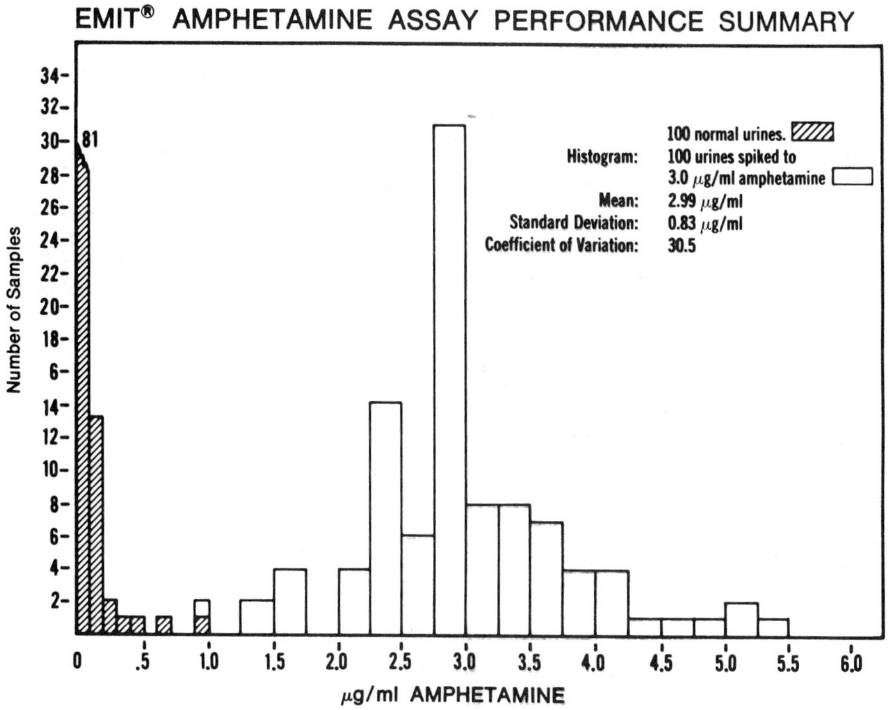

EMIT® AMPHETAMINE ASSAY PERFORMANCE SUMMARY

FIGURE 15.

TABLE 12

Effect of Operator Experience and Environment on EMIT Amphetamine Assay Results *

Operator experience (days)	Laboratory	Amphetamine concentration (μg/ml)**					Average deviation from mean
		1.5	2.0	3.0	5.0	8.0	
4	Syva	2.85	1.35	2.35	3.8	6.0	.45
7	West Coast	1.7	1.03	2.27	2.7	5.1	.78
14	West Coast	–	1.75	2.20	5.4	6.6	.37
30	East Coast	2.5	1.6	2.3	4.2	5.0	.44
60	Syva	1.5	1.55	2.2	8.9	6.6	1.08
Mean		2.14	1.46	2.26	5.00	5.86	
Standard deviation		0.64	0.28	0.06	2.38	0.78	

*One to four different urine samples were analyzed at each concentration by each operator. Average results are presented for all equal concentration samples.
**Spiked concentration.

Benzoyl Ecgonine (Cocaine Metabolite Assay)

Studies by Fish and Wilson[17] have shown that cocaine is rapidly hydrolyzed in vivo to benzoyl ecgonine. This compound is the principal urinary metabolite found in patients after cocaine abuse. The EMIT Benzoyl Ecgonine Assay detects principally this compound and slightly higher amounts of ecgonine. Cocaine is only poorly detected. No other compounds have been found that are detected by this assay. (See Table 13)

Preparation of the histogram shown in Figure 16 from 100 normal urines and 100 urines spiked with 1.6 μg/ml benzoyl ecgonine permits the selection of an appropriate cutoff value at 1.0 μg/ml. The data show that samples containing 1.6 μg/ml benzoyl ecgonine will assay for 1.6 ± .8 μg/ml greater than 95% of the time, and negative samples will assay below 0.4 μg/ml nearly all of the time.

Samples of pooled normal urine were spiked with benzoyl ecgonine at a level of 1.7 to 20.0 μg/ml. The samples were assayed by six different EMIT operators at different geographical locations to determine the precision of the assay as a function of the variables introduced by the technician and the different laboratory conditions. As

TABLE 13

EMIT Benzoyl Ecgonine Assay Response to Some Common Drugs

Detectability Limits

Drug	Typical concentrations in synthetic urine giving an EMIT reading equivalent to 1.0 μg/ml benzoyl ecgonine
Benzoyl ecgonine	1.0 μg/ml
Ecgonine	4.5 μg/ml
Cocaine	45.0 μg/ml
Caffeine	>1,000.0 μg/ml
Amphetamine	>1,000.0 μg/ml
Morphine	>1,000.0 μg/ml
Pentobarbital	>1,000.0 μg/ml
Secobarbital	>1,000.0 μg/ml
Phenobarbital	>1,000.0 μg/ml
Butabarbital	>1,000.0 μg/ml
Amobarbital	>1,000.0 μg/ml
Phenylpropanolamine	>1,000.0 μg/ml
Scopolamine	>1,000.0 μg/ml
Codeine	>1,000.0 μg/ml
Homatropine	>1,000.0 μg/ml
Atropine	>1,000.0 μg/ml
Prometazine	>1,000.0 μg/ml
Thorazine	>1,000.0 μg/ml
Methamphetamine	>1,000.0 μg/ml

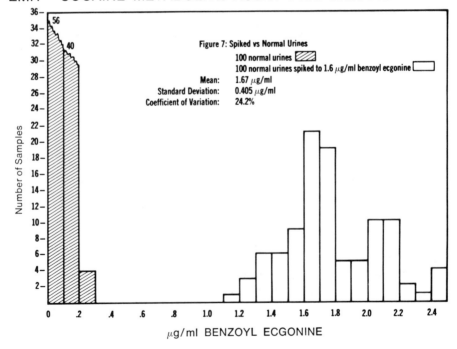

EMIT® COCAINE METABOLITE ASSAY PERFORMANCE SUMMARY

FIGURE 16.

TABLE 14

Benzoyl Ecgonine Assay Precision as a Function of Operator and Laboratory Location

Operator experience (days)	Laboratory	Benzoyl ecgonine concentration (μg/ml)							Average deviation from mean
		1.5	2.0	3.0	4.0	6.0	7.0	20.0	
1		1.3	1.5	2.6	2.9	5.4	4.8	13	0.81
1	East Coast	1.1	1.6	2.2	3.7	6.4	6.2	14	0.68
4	Syva	1.8	2.0	2.8	4.4	6.9	5.2	19	0.67
4	West Coast	1.8	2.2	3.0	3.8	5.2	7.0	20	0.70
8	South	1.5	2.5	2.5	5.0	7.2	7.2	26	1.73
36	Midwest	1.3	2.0	2.0	2.9	3.7	4.7	17	0.62
	Mean	1.47	1.97	2.5	3.8	5.8	5.9	18	
	Standard deviation	0.29	0.37	0.37	0.83	1.30	1.11	4.7	

in previous examples, all of the drug containing urines were correctly identified and, in addition, satisfactory quantitative precision was obtained between those participating in the study (see Table 14).

Review of Suggested Cutoff and Detection Levels for the EMIT Assay System

The five drug abuse classes which are detected by the EMIT system and the sensitivity of each assay are listed in Table 15. The detection levels and suggested cutoffs for each assay were determined from the histograms shown in the preceding sections in a manner completely analogous to that which was described in the FRAT assay discussion.

Clinical Results

In a performance study of the EMIT System, spiked urines were prepared from a pool of normal urines by the addition of a known quantity of from one to three drugs. Samples were labeled in a random fashion, frozen, and sent to EMIT testing centers throughout the United States.

Laboratory technicians with a variety of EMIT experience were instructed to assay each sample for opiates, barbiturates, amphetamines, and methadone. No operator had any prior knowledge of the contents of any of the samples. Of the six participating operators, none knew another's results.

Inspection of the experimental data (shown in the preceding sections dealing with assay per-

formance) indicates an excellent agreement between those participating in the study. The data demonstrate the reliability of the results regardless of operator training or geographic location, even when significant levels of other drugs are present. Qualitatively evaluation of all samples is shown in Table 16 using the following criteria to designate a positive sample:

Opiates	0.5 μg/ml or greater
Methadone	0.5 μg/ml or greater
Barbiturates	1.0 μg/ml or greater
Amphetamines	1.0 μg/ml or greater
Cocaine metabolite	1.0 μg/ml or greater

There were no errors for the opiates or methadone assays. Out of 595 total assays, there were only 7 or 1.2% incorrect results. Three false-negatives for barbiturates, three for amphetamines, and one cocaine metabolite false-positive were observed.

Conclusion

An enzyme immunoassay for opiates, barbiturates, methadone, amphetamine, and benzoyl ecgonine has been described in some detail. An advantage unique to the EMIT System is the immediacy of the assay result. The method requires no radioactive reagents, no incubation period, and offers specificity, quantification, and ease of sample manipulation. Since no sample pretreatment or incubation period is required, the results from an individual assay may be obtained a

TABLE 15

EMIT Drug Abuse Assays

EMIT assay	Drugs detected	Abuse drug assays cutoff level (μg/ml)	Detection level μg/ml
Opiates	Codeine		0.5
	Morphine	0.5	0.7
	Morphine glucuronide		1.25
	Heroin		7.7
Methadone	Methadone	0.5	0.7
	Alpha-acetylmethadol		4.0
Barbiturate	Secobarbital	1.0	2.0
	Phenobarbital		2.0
	Pentobarbital		3.5
	Amobarbital		3.5
	Butabarbital		1.0
	Thiopental		4.2
Amphetamine	Amphetamine	1.0	3.0
	Methamphetamine		2.0
Cocaine metabolite	Benzoyl ecgonine	1.0	1.6
	Ecgonine		4.5

TABLE 16

Qualitative Comparison of All Spiked Samples

	EMIT (+)	EMIT (−)
Spiked positives	253	6
Spiked negatives	1	335

few minutes after the sample is obtained from the operator. A prompt result is most desirable in hospital emergency rooms, law enforcement facilities, pre-employment screening, and methadone treatment programs.

Laboratories performing large numbers of urinalyses daily can utilize the EMIT System in one of the automated spectrometers (Gilford®, Abbott®) now commercially available. All of the sample manipulations necessary to perform an assay except sample addition can be automated on these instruments. Depending on instrument capabilities and laboratory demand up to 150 samples per hour can be analyzed.

APPENDIX 1

FRAT® OPIATE ASSAY

Signal Response Distribution from 100 Normal Negative Urine Samples And
the Same Urine Samples Spiked to a Level at 0.5 μg/ml Morphine

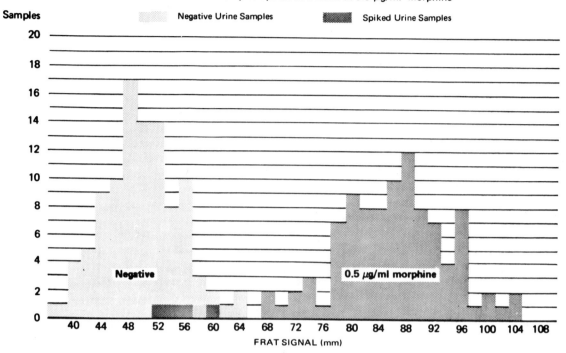

Histogram A.

FRAT® METHADONE ASSAY

Signal Response Distribution from 100 Normal Negative Urine Samples And
the Same Urine Samples Spiked to a Level at 0.5 μg/ml Methadone

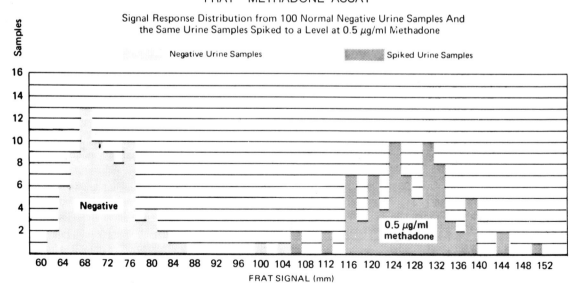

Histogram B.

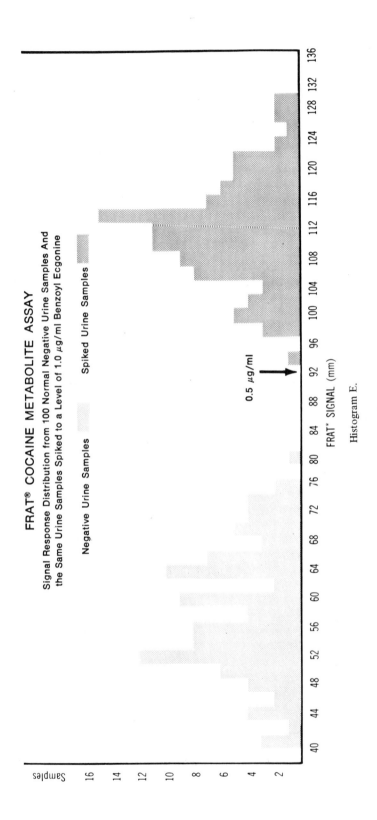

Histogram E.

Drug	Typical Concentrations in Synthetic Urine Giving a Signal Equivalent to 0.5 μg/ml Methadone	Relative Assay Response
Methadone	0.5 μg/ml	1.0000
Alpha-acetylmethadol	0.5 μg/ml	1.0000
Promethazine	30.0 μg/ml	0.0170
Dextromethorphan	155.0 μg/ml	0.0032
Chlorpromazine	160.0 μg/ml	0.0031
Meperidine	400.0 μg/ml	0.0001
Morphine	>500.0 μg/ml	<0.0001
Codeine	>500.0 μg/ml	<0.0001
Naloxone	>500.0 μg/ml	<0.0001
Dextropropoxyphene	>500.0 μg/ml	<0.0001

Histogram A.

Drug	Typical Concentrations in Synthetic Urine Giving a Signal Equivalent to 0.5 μg/ml Morphine	Relative Assay Response
Codeine	0.1 μg/ml	5.0000
Morphine	0.5 μg/ml	1.0000
Heroin	1.5 μg/ml	0.3300
Nalorphine	8.5 μg/ml	0.0590
Meperidine	35.0 μg/ml	0.0140
Diphenoxylate	90.0 μg/ml	0.0055
Dextromethorphan	165.0 μg/ml	0.0030
Chlorpromazine	255.0 μg/ml	0.0020
Naloxone	985.0 μg/ml	0.0005
Methadone	1000.0 μg/ml	<0.0005
Librium	>1000.0 μg/ml	<0.0005
Dextropropoxyphene	>1000.0 μg/ml	<0.0005

Histogram B.

Drug	Typical Concentrations in Synthetic Urine Giving a Signal Equivalent to 2.0 μg/ml Secobarbital	Relative Assay Response
Mephobarbital	0.8 μg/ml	2.50
Secobarbital	2.0 μg/ml	1.00
Phenobarbital	2.8 μg/ml	0.71
Pentobarbital	4.5 μg/ml	0.44
Amobarbital	6.8 μg/ml	0.29
Talbutal	7.6 μg/ml	0.26
Butabarbital	13.0 μg/ml	0.15
Thiopental	14.0 μg/ml	0.14
Glutethimide	25.0 μg/ml	0.08
Thimylal	40.0 μg/ml	0.05
Aprobarbital	46.0 μg/ml	0.04
Metharbital	200.0 μg/ml	0.01
Barbital	200.0 μg/ml	0.01
Probarbital	200.0 μg/ml	0.01

Histogram C.

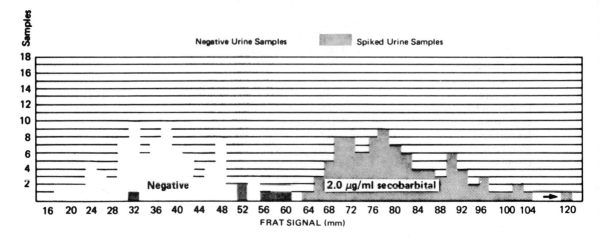

FRAT® BARBITURATE ASSAY

Signal Response Distribution from 100 Normal Negative Urine Samples And
the Same Urine Samples Spiked to a Level at 2.0 µg/ml Secobarbital

Histogram C.

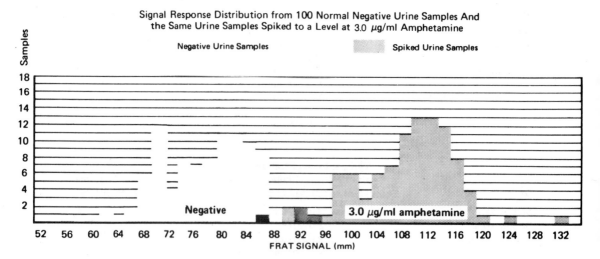

FRAT® AMPHETAMINE ASSAY

Signal Response Distribution from 100 Normal Negative Urine Samples And
the Same Urine Samples Spiked to a Level at 3.0 µg/ml Amphetamine

Histogram D.

Drug	Typical Concentrations in Synthetic Urine Giving a Signal Equivalent to 3.0 μg/ml Amphetamine	Relative Assay Response
Amphetamine	3.0 μg/ml	1.0000
Methamphetamine	4.4 μg/ml	0.6800
Mephentermine	5.6 μg/ml	0.5400
Phentermine	10.0 μg/ml	0.3000
Benzphetamine	35.0 μg/ml	0.0850
Cyclopentamine	45.0 μg/ml	0.0670
Phenmetrazine	50.0 μg/ml	0.0600
Ephedrine	70.0 μg/ml	0.0430
Phenylpropanolamine	75.0 μg/ml	0.0400
Nylidrin	90.0 μg/ml	0.0330
Methoxyphenamine	265.0 μg/ml	0.0110
Isoxsuprine	365.0 μg/ml	0.0080
Methylphenidiate	>1000.0 μg/ml	0.0030

Histogram D.

Drug	Typical Concentrations in Synthetic Urine Giving a Signal Equivalent to 1.0 μg/ml Benzoyl Ecgonine	Clinical Use
Benzoyl Ecgonine	1.0	Cocaine Metabolite
Ecgonine	12.0	Cocaine Metabolite
Cocaine	23.0	Local Anesthetic
Amphetamine	>1000.0	CNS Stimulant
Methadone	>1000.0	Narcotic Addiction
Morphine	>1000.0	Narcotic Analgesic
Pentobarbital	>1000.0	Sedative/Hypnotic
Secobarbital	>1000.0	Sedative/Hypnotic
Phenobarbital	>1000.0	Sedative/Hypnotic
Butabarbital	>1000.0	Sedative/Hypnotic
Amobarbital	>1000.0	Sedative/Hypnotic
Phenylpropanolamine	>1000.0	Antihistamine
Promethazine	>1000.0	Antihistamine
Codeine	>1000.0	Antitussive
Homatropine	>1000.0	Parasympatholytic
Atropine	>1000.0	Parasympatholytic
Scopolamine	>1000.0	Parasympatholytic

Histogram E.

REFERENCES

1. Spector, S. and Parker, C. W., Morphine radioimmunoassay, *Science,* 168, 1347, 1970.
2. Catlin, D. H., Cleeland, R., and Grunberg, E., A sensitive, rapid radioimmunoassay for morphine and immunologically related substances in urine and serum, *Clin. Chem.,* 19, 216, 1973.
3. Adler, F. L. and Lin, C. T., Detection of morphine by hemagglutination inhibition, *J. Immunol.,* 106, 1684, 1971.
4. Adler, F. L. Lin, C. T., and Catlin, D. H., Immunological studies on heroin addiction. I. Methodology and application of a hemagglutination inhibition test for detection of morphine, *Clin. Immunol. Immunopathol.,* 1, 53, 1972.
5. Rubenstein, K. E., Schneider, R. S., and Ullman, E. F., "Homogeneous" enzyme immunoassay. A new immunochemical technique, *Biochem. Biophys. Res. Commun.,* 47, 846, 1972.
6. Leute, R. K., Ullman, E. F., Goldstein, A., and Herzenberg, L. A., Spin immunoassay technique for determination of morphine, *Nature,* 236, 253, 1971.
7. Leute, R. K., Ullman, E. F., and Goldstein, A., Spin immunoassay of opiate narcotics in urine and saliva, *J.A.M.A.,* 221, 1231, 1972.

8. Van Weeman, B. K. and Schuurs, A. H. W. M., Immunoassay using antigen-enzyme conjugates, *Fed. Eur. Biochem. Soc. Lett.*, 15, 232, 1971.

9. Van Weeman, B. K. and Schuurs, A. H. W. M., Immunoassay using hapten-enzyme conjugates, *Fed. Eur. Biochem. Soc. Lett.*, 24, 77, 1972.

10 Engvall, E. and Perlmann, P., Enzyme-linked immunosorbent assay (ELISA) quantitative assay of immunoglobulin-G, *Immunochemistry*, 8, 871, 1971.

11. Engvall, E. and Perlmann, P., Enzyme-linked immunosorbent assay, ELISA, *J. Immunol.*, 109, 129, 1972.

12. Miedema, K., Boelhouwer, J., and Otten, J. W., Determination of proteins and hormones in serum by immunoassay using antigen-enzyme conjugates, *Clin. Chim. Acta*, 40, 187, 1972.

13. Way, E. L. and Adler, T. K., The biological disposition of morphine and its surrogates, *Bull. W.H.O.*, 25, 227, 1961.

14. For a general review, see Mulé, S. J., Methods for the analysis of narcotic analgesics and amphetamines, *J. Chromatogr. Sci.*, 10, 275, 1972.

15. Simon, E. J., Dole, W. P., and Hiller, J. M. Coupling of a new active morphine derivative to sepharose for affinity chromatography, *Proc. Natl. Acad. Sci.*, 69, 1835, 1972.

16. Beckett, A. H., Taylor, J. F., Casy, A. F., and Hassan, M. M. A., The biotransformation of methadone in man: Synthesis & identification of a major metabolite, *J. Pharm. Pharmacol.*, 20, 754, 1968.

17. Fish, F. and Wilson, W. D. C., Excretion of cocaine and its metabolites in man., *J. Pharm. Pharmacol.*, 21, 135, 1969.

18. Schneider, R. S., Lindquist, P., Wong, E., Ullman, E., and Rubinstein, K. E., Homogeneous enzyme immunoassay for opiates in urine, *Clin. Chem.*, 19, 821, 1973.

19. Finkle, B. S., Forsensic toxicology of drug abuse, *Anal. Chem.*, 44, 19A, 1972.

20. Baker, S. L., U.S. Army heroin abuse identification program in Vietnam: Implications for a methadone program. *Am. J. Public Health.*, 62, 857, 1972.

21. Valanju, N. N., Baden, M. M., Valanju, S. N., Mulligan, D., and Verma, S. K., Detection of biotransformed cocaine in urine from drug abusers. *J. Chromatogr.*, 81, 170, 1973.

GAS CHROMATOGRAPHIC MASS SPECTROMETRY IN
DRUG SCREENING BY IMMUNOASSAY

R. L. Hawks

TABLE OF CONTENTS

MASS SPECTROMETRY

From the time of its inception in the early part of the 20th century to the early 1950's, mass spectrometry was relegated principally to the realm of physicists. In the middle 1950's, the technique underwent increasing use by analytical and organic chemists which resulted in a cataclysmic effect in the areas of structural organic chemistry and analytical biochemistry.

The principles upon which the technique is based are quite simple. A molecule is introduced in the vapor phase into an ion source where it undergoes excitation, usually by electron bombardment, leading to a partial fragmentation of the molecule into a series of ionized fragments which can then be analyzed as to their ionic mass by passage through an ion separator. Figure 1 illustrates a general diagram of this type of system. The separator may function on the principle that, under a constant accelerating voltage, ion fragments will travel a certain linear distance at different velocities due to their different masses. The time-of-flight mass spectrometer is capable of providing a spectrum of such ions by precise measurement of the time required for a charged particle to traverse a specific distance. The time-of-flight instrument allows very rapid scan times but has relatively low resolution capabilities.

A second type of ion separator and the most widely used at present is the magnetic sector instrument, which operates on the principle that ions which are passed through a magnetic field will be deflected from a linear path as a function of their mass and velocity. The magnetic sector instrument provides high resolution.

The third type of separator in common use is the quadrupole separator. In this type of instrument, ionized fragments pass into an electrical field generated by DC and RF voltages applied simultaneously to a set of four metal rods, each about the size of a pencil, which are held in a square array. The alternating polarity electrostatic field thus generated gives bounded oscillations to an ion fragment of a given mass to charge ratio (m/e) and unbounded (collected and discharged on rods) oscillations to all other ions of different m/e. This type of system is physically less bulky than time-of-flight or magnetic sector instruments and is able to tolerate somewhat higher operating pressures. However, its resolution is generally inferior to a magnetic sector instrument.

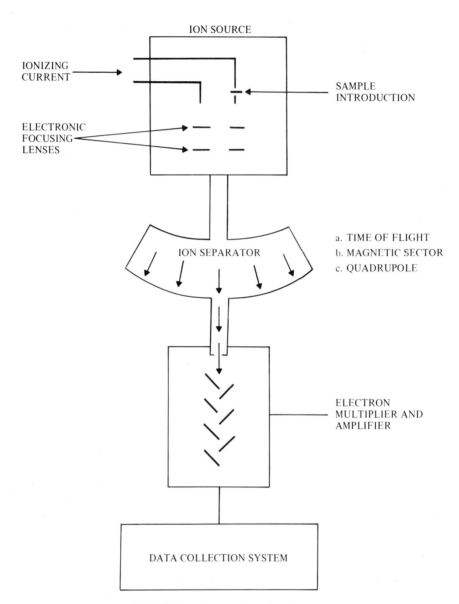

FIGURE 1.   Mass spectrometer diagram.

After the ionized particles are separated according to mass, they impinge on an electron multiplier, their signal is amplified, and the relative quantities of the ions are displayed by a recording device as a function of mass.

The spectrum of fragment ions and intensities thus acquired will be characteristic of structural features of the parent molecule. Figures 2b and 3b illustrate mass spectra of cocaine and methadone, respectively, obtained by electron impact fragmentation. Figures 2a and 3a illustrate the same compounds fragmented by another type of ionization known as chemical ionization.

The use of chemical ionization is a relatively new technique to mass spectrometrists and one that bears consideration in the area of drug research. A chemical ionization source differs from the usual electron impact source in that ionization of the molecule introduced to the source occurs by a more gentle process of chemical interaction with a charged reagent molecule such as CH_5^+ from methane. The CH_5^+ ion results from an electron impact excitation of methane gas which is introduced to the source. The CH_5^+ ions which are generated from the large excess of methane in the source then function as active chemical reagents

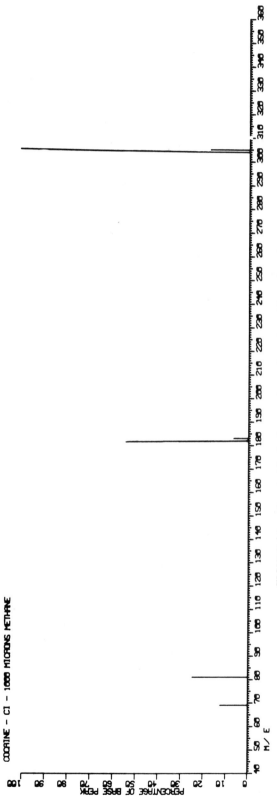

FIGURE 2A.   Chemical ionization spectrum of cocaine with methane ionization gas.

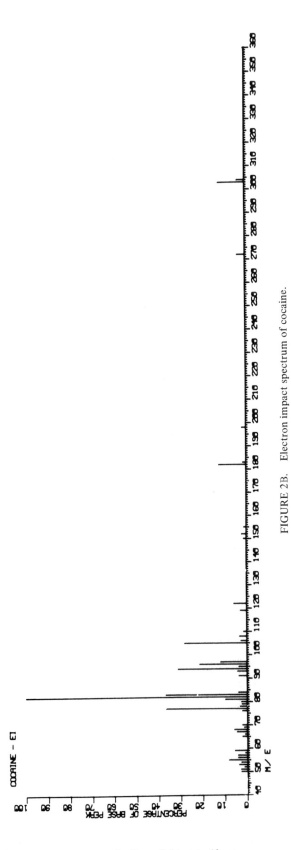

FIGURE 2B.   Electron impact spectrum of cocaine.

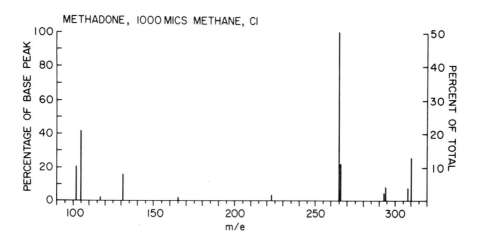

FIGURE 3A. Chemical ionization spectrum of methadone with methadone ionization gas.

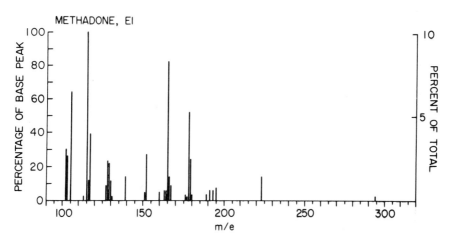

FIGURE 3B. Electron impact spectrum of methadone.

and react with the molecule to be fragmented by a process of proton transfer. This process results in a smaller amount of fragmentation and is particularly useful for certain drugs, such as the barbiturates,[1,2] which are sufficiently labile to electron impact to prevent any substantial formation of molecular ions. The difference in fragmentation pathways in the chemical ionization and electron impact modes is evident on comparison of the spectra in Figures 2 and 3. In Figure 2b, the cocaine molecule excited by electron impact yields a small molecular ion with a m/e of 303. It also yields ion fragments at m/e 272 and m/e 182 which arise from the fragmentation pathways shown in Figure 4. The major fragment ions of cocaine are lower molecular weight species at m/e

105 and smaller. The chemical ionization spectrum of cocaine (Figure 1a) shows little more than the molecular ion and the ion resulting from the loss of benzoic acid from the original structure. Chemical interaction between cocaine and a CH_5^+ ion from methane results in transfer of a proton to cocaine yielding the m/e 304 molecular ion, which then fragments under the influence of this higher energy state to give mainly the m/e 182 ion fragment. The smaller number of low-molecular-weight ion fragments in Figure 2a is indicative of the lower energy state of the molecule when it is excited by chemical ionization rather than by electron impact. Similar comparisons can be made on examination of the chemical ionization and electron impact spectra of methadone, which

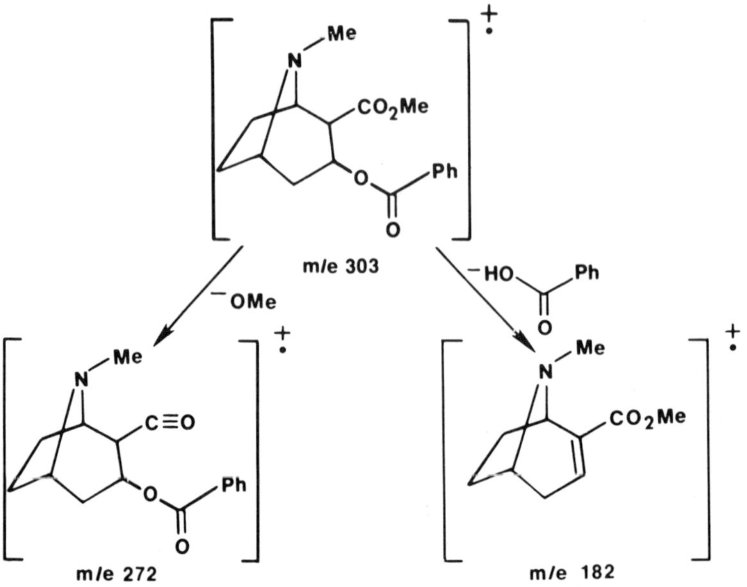

FIGURE 4. Fragmentation pathways of cocaine.

fragments along the pathways shown in Figure 5.

GAS CHROMATOGRAPHY

The development of gas-liquid chromatographic techniques is an extrapolation of the theories of paper partition chromatography. The gas chromatograph offers a powerful tool for the separation of complex mixtures and the quantitative analysis of their components. Separation is achieved by virtue of the fact that structurally different molecules will be absorbed into a thin film of viscous liquid with differing solubilities. A mixture of compounds is thus introduced to the end of a thin column which is packed with fine particles coated with a viscous liquid. A continuous stream of inert gas passes through the column and acts as a carrier for the molecules, which are in constant equilibrium between the gas phase and the viscous liquid phase. Since structurally different molecules will vary in their equilibrium between these two phases, the time required for traversing the length of the column will vary and separation of components is achieved. The effluent of the column is monitored by various types of detectors which might sense a component in the carrier gas by the component's effect on the conductivity of the gas as it is converted to ions (flame ionization detectors), by

its effect on the thermal conductivity of the carrier gas (thermal conductivity detectors), or by its ability to capture electrons whose flow in the detector generates a constant background current (electron capture detectors).

GAS CHROMATOGRAPHY-MASS SPECTROMETRY

The advantages of mating a gas chromatograph to a mass spectrometer to acquire structural data on small amounts of very pure effluents were obvious to early workers in analytical and biomedical chemistry when consideration was given to the fact that the sample quantities eluting from analytical gas chromatographic systems were similar to those quantities being introduced to mass spectrometers for structural analysis. In 1957, one of the first working systems was constructed by Holmes and Morrell[3] and was used to analyze low-molecular-weight components of city gas. The state of the art has dramatically improved since that early demonstration of the usefulness of gas chromatography-mass spectrometry (GC-MS). A major technical problem which arose early was the necessity of removing most of the carrier gas from the gas chromatograph effluent going into the ion source of the mass spectrometer. The ion source has to be operated at

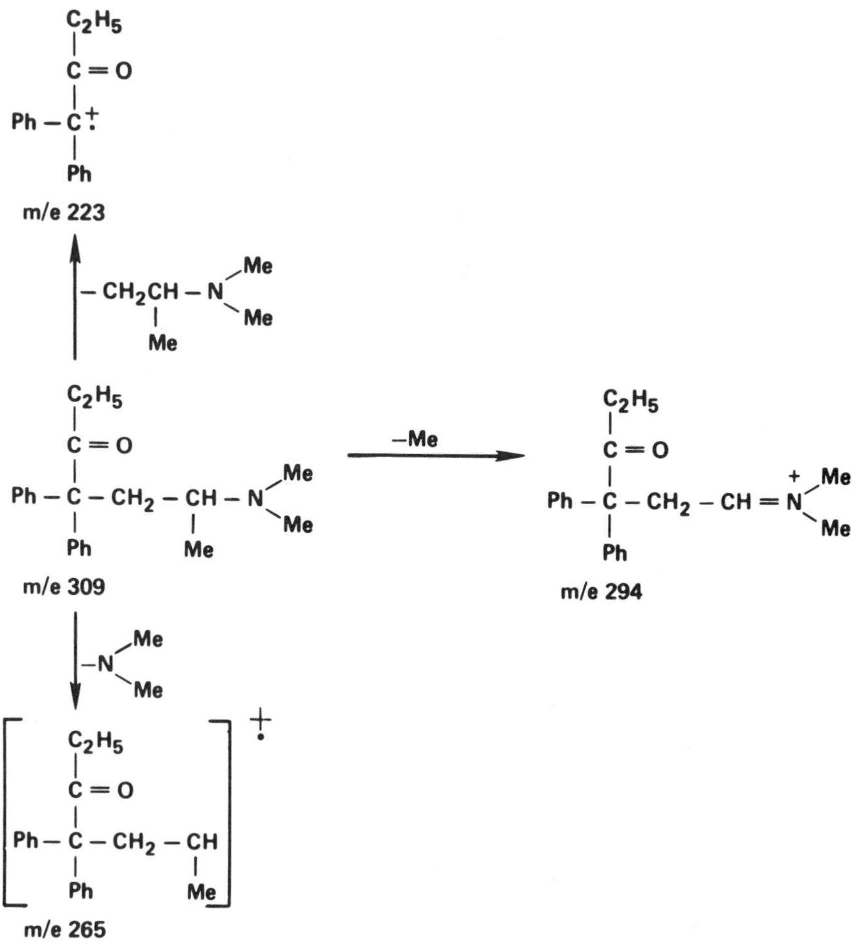

C_2H_5
$|$
$C = O$
$|$
$Ph - C \overset{+}{\cdot}$
$|$
Ph

m/e 223

$\uparrow$

$- CH_2CH - N \overset{Me}{\underset{Me}{\diagup}}$
$|$
Me

C_2H_5
$|$
$C = O$
$|$
$Ph - C - CH_2 - CH - N \overset{Me}{\underset{Me}{\diagup}}$
$|$ $\quad\quad\quad |$
$Ph \quad\quad\quad Me$

m/e 309

$\xrightarrow{-Me}$

C_2H_5
$|$
$C = O$
$|$
$Ph - C - CH_2 - CH = \overset{+}{N} \overset{Me}{\underset{Me}{\diagup}}$
$|$
Ph

m/e 294

$\downarrow -N \overset{Me}{\underset{Me}{\diagup}}$

$\left[\begin{array}{c} C_2H_5 \\ | \\ C = O \\ | \\ Ph - C - CH_2 - CH \\ | \quad\quad\quad | \\ Ph \quad\quad\quad Me \end{array} \right]^{\overset{+}{\cdot}}$

m/e 265

FIGURE 5. Fragmentation pathways of methadone.

relatively low pressures and cannot ordinarily tolerate a large gas input. Various types of separators have been designed which remove very low-molecular-weight (carrier gas) material from the effluent prior to its introduction to the ion source. Considerable concentration enrichment of the compounds to be analyzed is thus achieved. The reader is referred to a recent review if more details on types of separators are desired.[4] A diagram of a hypothetical GC-MS system is illustrated in Figure 6. The various data-processing functions will be discussed below.

Under favorable conditions, a modern GC-MS system can provide a mass spectral identification from as little as 0.1 picogram of material. The GC-MS system offers a method of acquiring rapid structural information in metabolism studies. Since most biotransformations involve simple structural changes such as hydrolysis of an ester group (cocaine),[5] hydroxylation (THC)[6,7] or N-dimethylation (acetylmethadol or methadone),[8,9] the structural changes are usually immediately apparent from a mass spectrum of the metabolite. An increase in mass of 16 atomic mass units (amu) is indicative of hydroxylation, a decrease in mass of 14 amu is indicative of demethylation, and so forth. Due to the sensitivity inherent in the method, the sample quantities of metabolites which can be eluted from analytical thin-layer chromatograms are sufficient for complete fragmentation analysis. The use of GC-MS as a powerful analytical tool is a rapidly growing field.[10-12]

Present systems have the capability of being focused at particular m/e values, rather than scanning the whole spectrum of ions, and thus

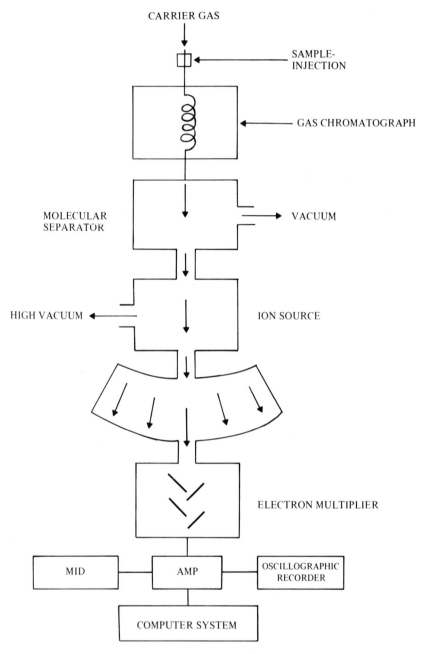

CARRIER GAS

SAMPLE-
INJECTION

GAS CHROMATOGRAPH

MOLECULAR
SEPARATOR

VACUUM

HIGH VACUUM

ION SOURCE

ELECTRON MULTIPLIER

MID

AMP

OSCILLOGRAPHIC
RECORDER

COMPUTER SYSTEM

FIGURE 6.   Gas chromatograph—mass spectrometer diagram.

provide a constant monitor for particular fragments. When used in this manner, sensitivity is
considerably enhanced due to the favorable time-
averaging of the signal; integration time at a given
spectral position is much increased over the time
spent there in a normal scan. Thus, the mass
spectrometer is functioning essentially as a single
fragment detector for the gas chromatograph.

By focusing on the principal fragment of a
given compound, it becomes possible to provide a
gas chromatogram of that material in the low
picogram range. By simultaneously introducing
into the gas chromatograph an internal standard
(preferably a heavy atom derivative of the
molecule in question) along with the unknown
material and feeding this second signal to a second

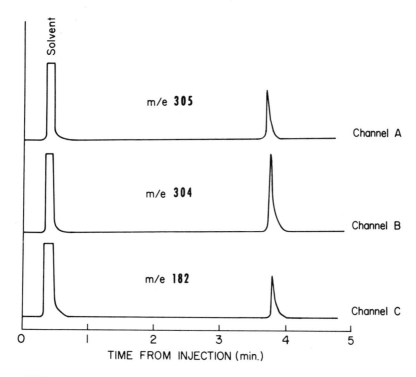

FIGURE 7.   Mass fragmentography of cocaine using d₁-cocaine internal standard.

strip chart recorder channel, a means is provided to quantitate the unknown. If more specificity for a given molecular structure is desired in the case, for instance, where two compounds might have similar retention times on the gas chromatograph as well as the same principal fragment, then an additional fragment of the unknown molecule can be monitored by the mass spectrometer and the signal fed into a third channel of a strip chart recorder. This then provides two gas chromatograms (one for each monitored fragment) of the same molecule from the same sample injection. The ratios of the intensities of the peaks provided for the two fragments on the two chromatograms will be similar to the ratio of the peaks for these fragments in the usual mass spectrum of the material.

Figure 7 illustrates the type of chromatograms resulting from a fragmentography procedure where two principal fragments of cocaine generated by chemical ionization were monitored relative to an internal standard of mono-deuterated cocaine. Channel *a* is tuned to monitor the m/e 305 peak of the deuterated standard and channels *b* and *c* the m/e 304   and m/e 182 of the unknown cocaine. The peaks are coincident in gas chromatographic

retention time since they all derive from the cocaine molecule. Since the quantity of standard (deuterated cocaine) giving rise to the 305 peak in channel *a* is known, the amount of cocaine in the sample is determined by comparison of this peak with that in channel *b*. Further confidence in the specificity of the analysis is achieved by comparing the ratio of the 303 and 182 peaks. This ratio should correspond with that from the standard spectra of cocaine (Figure 2a) if no interfering ion fragments are present in either channel at this particular retention time. It is highly unlikely that any interfering substance could coincidentally manifest the same retention time as well as the same two principal mass fragments in the same ratio as the molecule in question; a very specific analytical tool is thus provided.

Commercial GC-MS sytems offer a wide variety of data-handling packages. The simplest output display is the rapid-scanning oscillographic recorder, which provides a mass spectral display of peaks at several different amplifications simultaneously. The operator is required to measure individual peaks in order to normalize the entire spectrum to a 100% base peak. The possibility always exists, of course, of introducing too much sample and thus saturating even the lowest amplification scale. The sample level is generally empirically determined where a variety of substance types and concentrations are handled. Data-handling efficiency is increased by employing an analog-to-digital interface between the mass spectrometer output and a small digital computer programmed to acquire and store the data. These programs are capable of presenting the data via a mechanical printer or teletype in a variety of forms. They automatically normalize data and give a printout of the mass spectrum in terms of relative percentages. Auxillary components can be purchased for various brands of mass spectrometers which adapt them specifically for quantitative use. Units for magnetic sector instruments offer a means of switching between two or three accelerating voltages, thus providing a means of passing two or three specific fragments through the instruments' fixed slits. Another type of unit for multiple ion detection is actually an analog computer system which sets the specific DC/RF voltage on a quadrupole-type instrument necessary to pass particular fragments through the quadrupole separator. This system also feeds the signals from the electron multiplier to a series of strip chart recorders, each pen recorder receiving the signal generated by a particular fragment.

For purposes of quantitative use, the quadrupole-type instrument seems to offer some advantages over the magnetic sector type. In general, the latter provides more resolution, but high resolution is usually not a major requirement in an analytical instrument. The principal advantage of the quadrupole instrument for multiple ion detection is its ability to be focused at specific ion fragments over its entire spectral range where a magnetic sector instrument is limited to a variation of 20 to 50% of its total range. Another advantage of the quadrupole system is its tolerance for higher operating pressures than magnetic sector instruments, about 10^{-5} torr as compared to about 10^{-6} torr for the latter. Higher operating pressures allow more carrier gas to be introduced to the source, and consequently less critical efficiency is required of the molecular separator. More carrier gas in the source also yields a higher quantity of reagent ions with a subsequent boost to efficiency of ionization in the case of chemical ionization sources. Further details of comparison of the types of GC-MS

systems as well as applications may be found in recent reviews.[10],[11]

Cost is of major consideration in the acquisition of a GC-MS system to any analytical process. A useful system will cost from $30,000 upwards and will require experienced scientific personnel to run it. A GC-MS system which is available for use by several laboratories on a shared basis is a means of making the technique available to many laboratories which could not otherwise support such a system.

It should be emphasized that a GC-MS system, due to its complexity, can be assumed to involve more "down-time" than other types of instrumental analytical systems. The decision to acquire such a system should involve consideration of the technical expertise necessary for the function of the system. Training is often provided by the manufacturers of GC-MS equipment. A selected list of GC-MS manufacturers and instrument specifications appears in Table 1.

RADIOIMMUNOASSAY

In recent years, we have seen a rapid growth in the use of immunoassay techniques in drug-screening laboratories where large numbers of samples are required to be processed cheaply and rapidly with a high degree of sensitivity and reliability. However, certain inherent limitations of the immunoassay methods should be noted, particularly in view of their expanding role in forensic analysis. The most significant limitation of immunoassay is that of cross-reacting substances that can interfere in the antibody-antigen reaction. Regardless of the type of immunoassay used, one is monitoring an interaction between an antigenic molecule and an antibody protein whose surface has structural characteristics at certain places which allows a binding between the antigen and the antibody protein. The extent to which this "receptor site" on the antibody is specific for the particular antigenic molecule in question is a function of the structural nature of the haptenic species used to produce the antibody as well as to a myriad of conditions of animal species, inoculation, time course of treatment and to the methods of purification of antibody serum. Regardless of the care involved in preparing a highly specific antibody substance for immunoassay, the final product at best can only be considered as a "highly specific" species but not a unique one.

TABLE 1

Manufacturers and Characteristics of Selected Commercial Gas Chromatograph-Mass Spectrometer Systems

Manufacturer	Model	Instrument type	Approximate mass range (amu)	Approximate resolving power
AEI Scientific Apparatus, Inc. 3 Corporate Park Drive White Plains, New York 10605	MS-30 MS-902	Magnetic sector Magnetic sector	1–2,400 1–7,200	10,000 100,000
Aero Vac Corporation P.O. Box 448 Troy, New York 12181	270 Series	Magnetic sector	70 to 500	35 to 250
Bendix Corporation 1775 Mt. Read Boulevard Rochester, New York 14603	MA2 MA3	Time of flight Time of flight	1,200 600	700 300
Du Pont/CEC E.I. du Pont de Nemours & Co., Inc. 1500 South Shamrock Avenue Monrovia, California 91016	21-104 21-490 21-491 21-492 21-621	Magnetic sector Magnetic sector Magnetic sector Magnetic sector Quadrupole	1–2,000 2–2,400 2–2,400 1–4,000 1–300	2,500 1,100 2,500 15,000 2X Mass no.
Electronic Associates, Inc. 4151 Middlefield Road Palo Alto, California 94303	QUAD 160 QUAD 300	Quadrupole Quadrupole	1–300 1–800	Unit resolution Unit resolution
Extranuclear Laboratories, Inc. P.O. Box 11512 Pittsburgh, Pennsylvania 15238	S-350 S-500 S-1,400 S-3,000	Quadrupole Quadrupole Quadrupole Quadrupole	0–350 0–500 0–1,400 0–3,000	1,600 1,500 1,200 1,000
Finnigan Corporation 595 North Pastoria Avenue Sunnyvale, California 94086	1015 3000	Quadrupole Quadrupole	1–750 10–500	R = M R = M
Hewlett-Packard 1601 California Avenue Palo Alto, California 94304	5930A	Quadrupole	0–65°	Unit resolution
Lexington Instruments Corporation 241 Crescent Street Waltham, Massachusetts 02154	RMS-11	Magnetic sector	2–200	70
LKB Instruments, Inc. 12221 Parklawn Drive Rockville, Maryland 20852	LKB-9,000	Magnetic sector	2–2,000	5,000
Nuclide 642 East College Avenue State College, Pennsylvania 16801	12-90-G	Magnetic sector	1–6,000	10,000
Perkin-Elmer Corporation 723G Main Avenue Norwalk, Connecticut 06852	RMS-4 RMU-6L	Magnetic sector Magnetic sector	1–1,200 1–4,000	2,500 10,000
Process Instruments 1943 Broadway Brooklyn, New York 11207	M-60	Magnetic sector	1–360	1 at 250

TABLE 1 (continued)

Manufacturers and Characteristics of Selected Commercial Gas Chromatograph-Mass Spectrometer Systems

Manufacturer	Model	Instrument type	Approximate mass range (amu)	Approximate resolving power
Quinton Instruments 3051 44th Avenue West Seattle, Washington 98199	M3[c,d]	Magnetic sector	2–140	50
Scientific Research Instruments Corp. 6707 Whitestone Road Baltimore, Maryland 21207	MS-8[c] MR-2[c] CHEMSPECT-QUAD CQ-4	Magnetic sector Magnetic sector Quadrupole with chemical ionization source	10–60 1–64 1–400	30 100 350
Thompson-CSF 51, Boulevard de le Republique 78 Chatou, France	TSN-215M[c] ex SM-100R[c] TSN-206C	Magnetic sector Magnetic sector	Multicollector masses 4, 28, 32, 40, 44 1–3,000	100 at 1% ≥10,000 up to 15,000
Varian Associates 611 Hansen Way Palo Alto, California 94303	CH5 CH7 MAT111	Magnetic sector Magnetic sector Magnetic sector	1–3,600 1–3,600 1–1,000	10,000 5,000 1,000

Receptor sites are not likely rigid structural species but, rather, are somewhat labile groups of chemical moieties whose stereochemical orientations are such that they can effectively interact with compatible binding features of the antigenic molecules. This implies the probability of several antigenic species with a high affinity for a specific site. Obviously, certain structural and stereochemical features must be common to these antigens to allow binding at the same receptor site. The usual means of determining specificity is to choose molecules of similar structure to that one to which the antibody was raised and to observe the extent of their reaction with the antibody. This empirical approach suffers from certain drawbacks. Specific structures for cross-reactivity testing are chosen on the basis of their structural and stereochemical similarity to the antigenic molecule. The thoroughness of this testing regimen is a function of the experience and the subjective judgment of the researcher. Often a substance which on paper shows little structural similarity to the antigen and is thus overlooked as a cross-reactive species will interfere and may escape detection. An example is the significant cross-reactivity of diphenylhydantonin[13] and diazepam[14] with thyroxine in the latter's protein-binding assay. The stereochemical-structural similarity of these two compounds to thyroxine became evident only after examination of the three structures by X-ray crystallography.

The problem of potential cross-reactivity in immunoassay systems can be minimized by the application of GC-MS instrumentation as a complementary tool. GC-MS systems are among the few analytical systems which offer sensitivity of an order similar to immunoassay methods; at the same time, they incorporate a much higher degree of specificity, as discussed earlier. GC-MS systems focused on specific mass fragments of molecules monitored as column effluents from a gas chromatographic column are capable of detecting material in the low picogram range and can provide for that material a gas chromatographic retention time, coincidental monitoring of several fragments from the same molecule along with the approximate intensity ratios of those fragments. The probability of the presence of an interfering substance in a biological sample which manifests coincidentally these same characteristics is most unlikely except in the case of stereoisomer.

Consider a radioimmunoassay which is to be

applied to the analysis of several hundred samples daily in which the desired analytical result is a positive or negative indication of the presence of morphine in the sample. A positive result of the procedure would give rise to an observed radioactivity in a sample in excess of that found in drug-free controls. The question of how much of an observed difference in activity will constitute a positive analysis is one which needs careful consideration in terms of the potential for unknown interferences and human error in the analysis. As the antibody becomes more specific, these lower limits can be established with increasing confidence although this confidence can sometimes be detrimental if one succumbs to the fallacious assumption that the antibody is unique for the particular drug in question. By simultaneously analyzing by GC-MS a portion of the samples being carried through the immunoassay screen, a very effective quality control is provided. If the portion chosen to be analyzed by GC-MS includes both a random sampling and those positive results of the immunoassay which occur near its lower confidence limits, a check is provided on systematic errors which may occur in the immunoassay as well as a check on those results which are more likely to be reported as false positives. The overall effect of this quality control is such as to lower the limits of the immunoassay procedure within which one has a given confidence in the report of a positive result.

The use of the GC-MS system as a confirmatory tool for positive analyses from a radioimmunoassay procedure has obvious advantages over gas chromatography alone, thin-layer chromatography or microcrystallography. All of these techniques can be considered as absolute analytical tools only in their ability to yield a negative result. The absence of a peak with a given retention time, a spot with a particular R_f or a crystal of appropriate structure in the three methods is an absolute indication of the absence of the compound in question assuming that due consideration is given to the methods' limits of sensitivity. The presence of any or all of these characteristics can only be considered as circumstantial evidence of the presence of the compound. The question of interfering substances is never completely removed by any of these methods, particularly in borderline cases where confirmation in one method cannot be duplicated in another because of sensitivity limits. GC-MS provides specificity and sensitivity sufficient to make a confirmation of this type much more certain. This sort of certainty becomes quite important in prosecution cases for drug offenses and in the controversial area of immunoassay procedures as screens to detect drug use in present or prospective employees in private industry.

One of the most useful applications of GC-MS for the immunoassay researcher is in the area of biotransformation and disposition of drugs. It is most important to have knowledge of the metabolism of a drug so as to be able to predict the relative concentrations of the drug and its metabolites in the biological fluid to be assayed. A considerable amount of time and effort is required to prepare and test an antibody for an immunoassay. It becomes critical to be certain that the antigen in question is the appropriate metabolic manifestation of the drug to be analyzed. For an optimum assay, one needs to be sure he is considering the species of greatest concentration in the biological medium in question. An immunoassay screening for cocaine in urine, for example, would be of very limited use if the antibody recognized only cocaine itself and not one or both of its urinary metabolic forms, benzoylecgonine or ecgonine.[5] Slight metabolic structural changes in molecules have profound effects on the way the molecule will react to an antibody. GC-MS offers a useful means of investigating these transformations prior to forming the antibody.

In summary, the usefulness of GC-MS in immunoassay screening and development is obvious and will undoubtedly be used to a greater extent in this field in the near future as immunoassay techniques become more widespread and the consequences of their results become more significant.

REFERENCES

1. **Fales, H. M., Milne, G. W. A., and Axenrod, T.,** Identification of barbiturates by chemical ionization mass spectrometry, *Anal. Chem.,* 42, 1432, 1970.

2. **Fales, H. M., Milne, G. W. A., and Colburn, R. W.,** Chemical ionization mass spectrometry of complex molecules. X. Biogenetic amines, *Anal. Chem.,* 45, 1952, 1973.

3. **Holmes, J. C. and Morrell, F. A.,** Oscillographic mass spectrometric monitoring of gas chromatography, *Appl. Spectrosc.,* 11, 86, 1957.

4. **Ryhage, R. and Wikstrom, S.,** Gas chromatography-mass spectrometry, in *Mass Spectrometry: Techniques and Applications,* Milne, G. W. A., Ed., Wiley-Interscience, New York, 1971, 91.

5. **Fish, F. and Wilson, W. D. C.,** Excretion of cocaine and its metabolites in man, *J. Pharm. Pharmacol.,* 21 (Suppl.), 135 S, 1969.

6. **Wall, M. E., Brine, D. R., Brine, G., Pitt, C. G., Freudenthal, R. I., and Christensen, H. D.,** Isolation, structure, and biological activity of several metabolites of Δ^9-tetrahydrocannabinol, *J. Am. Chem. Soc.,* 92, 3466, 1970.

7. **Pitt, C. G., Hauser, F., Hawks, R. L., Sathe, S., and Wall, M. E.,** The synthesis of 11-hydroxy-Δ^9-tetrahydrocannabinol and other physiologically active metabolites of Δ^8- and Δ^9-tetrahydrocannabinol, *J. Am. Chem. Soc.,* 94, 8578, 1972.

8. **Pohland, A., Sullivan, H. R., and Lee, H. M.,** Analgesics. Des-N-methyl methadone analogs, *Proceedings of the 136th Annual Meeting of the Am. Chem. Soc.,* 15-0, 1959.

9. **Pohland, A., Boaz, H. E., and Sullivan, H. R.,** Synthesis and identification of metabolites resulting from the biotransformation of *DL*-methadone in man and in the rat, *J. Med. Chem.,* 14, 194, 1971.

10. **Junk, G. A.,** Gas chromatograph-mass spectrometer combinations and their applications, *Int. J. Mass Spectrom. Ion Phys.,* 8, 1, 1972.

11. **Waller, G. R.** *Biochemical Applications of Mass Spectrometry,* Wiley-Interscience, New York, 1972.

12. **Brooks, C. J. W.,** Gas chromatography-mass spectrometry, *Mass Spectrom.,* 1, 288, 1971.

13. **Wolff, J., Standaert, M., and Rall, J. E.,** Thyroxine displacement from serum proteins and depressions of serum protein-bound iodine by certain drugs, *J. Clin. Invest.,* 40, 1373, 1961.

14. **Schussler, G.,** Diazepam competes for thyroxine binding sites, *J. Pharmacol. Exp. Ther.,* 178, 204, 1971.

DISCUSSION

Each of the foregoing presentations (Drs. Gross, Spector, Adler, and VanVunakis) stimulated general discussions by all of the participants. The following is a summary of these discussions in which no attempt is made to identify the discussant, but rather to emphasize those points that appeared to be of general interest.

There was considerable discussion concerning specificity. As noted in the presentations, there is general agreement about the variations in specificity from animal to animal and bleeding to bleeding. One of the more important variations is the ability or the lack of it for antisera to recognize morphine glucuronide. It is desirable to use antisera that will be sensitive to the glucuronide if the assay is intended to ascertain the use of morphine or heroin. In determining the sensitivity to morphine glucuronide, the question was raised as to what is actually being measured. In some instances, the glucuronide used was that actually isolated from urine and purified. In other cases, it was determined indirectly by measuring morphine before and after acid hydrolysis of the sample.

This raised a discussion concerning whether there was any degradation of morphine during acid hydrolysis. Although some investigators felt that some degradation does occur, it was admitted that there are little hard data to support this. Some of the experiences may vary due to different conditions. Using a 1:10 dilution of concentrated hydrochloric acid in an autoclave for 20 min, very little degradation of morphine is claimed, whereas boiling the urine with dilute acid for 60 min appears to produce some differences that may be attributed to partial destruction of morphine. It is not known if such suspected degradation products will react with the antisera or not.

There are obviously a number of methods employed to separate the hapten-antibody complex from the free hapten prior to counting. Some experiences with charcoal or dextran-coated charcoal were described. Although this procedure offers some advantages, e.g., rapidity, it was felt to be too harsh, because it will disturb the equilibrium of free to bound hapten and often "strips" the antibody of hapten. The ammonium sulfate method presents a similar problem, as the introduction of high ionic strength requires an antibody with relatively high affinity for the hapten. In the case of morphine, the equilibrium of free to bound hapten is further complicated by the fact that the marker molecule, the labeled hapten, is usually either dihydromorphine or iodinated morphine. In general, it was recognized that the nitrocellulose filter technique was perhaps the gentlest technique for separating antibody-bound hapten.

A solid phase method was also described. In this approach, the antisera is coated onto polystyrene cups, which may be frozen and stored until use. The sample containing the drug and the marker are added, the cups incubated, the supernatant removed, and the contents counted by dissolution of the cups in the scintillation solvent. The method may be easily automated.

Another simplification of the separation step using a solid phase technique was described. In this method an acrylamide gel is used to bind the antibody and after the addition of the reagents directly to the scintillation vial, it is shaken and allowed to set, and the radioactivity determined following precipitation. The geometry of the scintillation counter is such that only the labeled material in the supernatant is counted. Several participants pointed out that, in general, they have had considerable difficulty in obtaining reproducible results by counting the supernatant. This was particularly true when ammonium sulfate is used as a certain amount of coprecipitation occurs.

Another area that was discussed at length concerned the pharmacokinetics of the drugs, particularly morphine, as followed by immunoassays. The practical question to be answered is how long after a single dose of morphine or heroin can the drug be detected in the blood or urine. Obviously the most sensitive method should detect drug or its metabolite for the longest time interval. There were some feelings expressed that unknown products, presumed metabolites, were being detected in urine of addicts after heroin use. As the absolute (total) metabolism of heroin or morphine is not known, a considerable amount of research remains to be done in this area. On the other hand, for screening purposes, it is only necessary to detect morphine equivalents.

It was pointed out that although it is possible to prepare rather specific antisera by gel permeation chromatography, its value has to be balanced against its higher cost, plus the fact that all positive results require corroboration anyway.

There was an extensive discussion on the EMIT

system. Such questions as how the enzyme activity is influenced by steric factors involved in connecting the determinant hapten to the enzyme remain to be answered. It is known, however, that there is an optimum length for the "leash" — the connecting linkage between the hapten and enzyme. Apparently, the hapten is bound to a reactive site near the enzyme active site(s), but if the leash is too long, when the enzyme binds with the antibody, the active site on the enzyme is not blocked. On the other hand, if the leash is too short, the repulsive forces between the two macromolecules will make binding difficult. It was pointed out that there is also a limit to the size of the molecule that can be used as the hapten, and to date this approach has only worked with drug molecules, i.e., about the size of steroids.

Another aspect of the EMIT, and to some extent FRAT, system that was of interest was that it is not an equilibrium system but a competitive reaction. Only enough time is allowed to permit thermal equilibrium, so that the control and final readings are made within one minute. This tends to create problems when the concentration of the hapten is low, as it takes a finite period of time for the hapten molecules to "find" the binding sites on the antibody.

It was brought out that attempts to carry out immunoassay procedures on old urine samples can present problems. Although the ionic strength is not critical, old urines tend to have a relatively high pH due to the formation of ammonia. In the case of EMIT, it was recommended that urines a few days old, stored without a preservative or no refrigeration should have their pH checked and adjusted prior to analysis. The presence of lysozymes and complement proteins in serum requires that these be removed before the analysis. Crab shells may be used to remove lysozyme, but denaturing by heating is required for the proteins. This means using a 200 microliter sample of the serum to ensure having sufficient material, although only 50 microliters are actually needed.

There was interest expressed in the development of a multiple antibody assay that would measure three to five drugs at the same time. It was noted that some efforts are being made along this line, e.g., a RIA kit for morphine and barbiturates, is in the final stages of testing.

EVALUATION OF IMMUNOASSAYS FOR THE DETECTION OF DRUGS SUBJECT TO ABUSE

EVALUATION AND CLINICAL APPLICATION OF THE IMMUNOASSAYS FOR MORPHINE

D. H. Catlin

TABLE OF CONTENTS

INTRODUCTION

Recognition of the increased use and abuse of drugs has created a demand for improved methodology for the detection of these drugs and their metabolites in human biological fluids. Initially, the demand was met by familiar methods such as thin-layer chromatography (TLC) and gas chromatography (GC), and to a lesser extent by spectrofluorometry. Procedures based on these techniques usually include a separation procedure involving an extraction or absorption followed by concentration of the extract or eluate. Many laboratories include a hydrolysis step in order to convert morphine glucuronide, the major urinary metabolite of heroin and morphine,[1] into free morphine. Since these steps contribute significantly to the complexity of the procedure and the analysis time, numerous modifications and improvements have recently been developed. Some of these developments have been reviewed in this volume or are described elsewhere.[2-13]

A major contribution to the detection of drugs has been the recent application of the classical principles of immunoassay to the problem of identification and measurement of these drugs and/or other metabolites in body fluids. Since Spector and Parker described a procedure for producing antibodies specific for morphine by the immunization of a rabbit with a hapten-protein conjugate, carboxy-methylmorphine-bovine serum albumin,[22] there has been a proliferation of articles applying the same principles to other drugs of abuse: barbiturates,[32] methadone,[19] mescaline,[33] and pentazocine.[34] Currently, four different immunoassays for morphine are commercially available: free-radical assay technique (FRAT);* enzyme-multiplied immunoassay technique (EMIT);* hemagglutination-inhibition;** and radioimmunoassay.*** The basic principles and procedures of these assays are described in other chapters in this book and elsewhere.[14-25]

It is generally recognized that immunoassays are superior to the classical chromatography tech-

*Manufactured by Syva Corporation, 3181 Porter Drive, Palo Alto, California 94304.
**Distributed by R. D. Products, P.O. Box E, Victor, New York 14564.
***Manufactured by Roche Diagnostics, Hoffmann-LaRoche,

niques with respect to the critical parameters of sensitivity, rapidity of analysis, and simplicity. They permit a high ratio of analyses/analyst and are amenable to automation. The availability of the immunoassays has created a demand for comparative data assessing their performance and for information concerning their proper interpretation and applications in the analysis of biological samples for drugs of abuse. The purpose of this paper is to present concepts pertinent to the evaluation of the immunoassays for morphine, to summarize the clinical data obtained to compare the performance of three different immunoassays for morphine, and to present guidelines for the application of immunoassays to detection of drugs of abuse as well as to the proper interpretation of their results.

DEFINITIONS

Prior to discussing either the comparative performance data or the applications, it is necessary to define a number of terms. While many of these terms are familiar in the context of the nonserological assays, their use with reference to the immunoassays requires amplification.

Sensitivity

Sensitivity is the lowest concentration of a compound which can be detected in undiluted body fluid. Often it is referred to as the "detection limit" or "cutoff level." With respect to the immunoassays, sensitivity is a function of the particular antiserum or pooled antiserum used in the assay, the concentration of antiserum, and the amount of labeled drug or antigen. For most immunoassays, the results are expressed in numerical terms, that is, the data are continuous. Accordingly the sensitivity can be selected at any concentration which exceeds a particular minimum value. This value is established experimentally by determining the range and frequency distribution of results obtained from the analysis of samples submitted by individuals known not to be receiving the drug. The sensitivity is selected to exceed any desired fraction of the frequency distribution of results on normal samples. The manufacturers or distributors of the immunoassays usually recommend a sensitivity, more commonly, the value is determined by the experience of a laboratory with a particular assay, or by those individuals who receive and interpret the test results. Sensitivities between 0.05 and 0.50 μg/ml are readily achieved by the immunoassays for morphine.

Specificity

Specificity is the degree to which an assay can distinguish one compound from another. For the immunoassays, specificity is a function of the particular population of antibody molecules contained in the antiserum. In turn, the specificity of an antiserum is in part a function of the particular antigen used to immunize the animal. In accordance with the known heterogeneity of antibodies, each bleeding from an immune animal is a unique reagent. Accordingly, one may anticipate that the specificity of an immunoassay for morphine or any other drug may vary between immunoassay manufacturers and within reagent lots supplied by the same manufacturer.

Considering only those immunoassays for morphine which are commercially available at the present time, it is recognized that compounds other than free morphine (for example, dextromethorphan,[23] poppy seed metabolites,[15] and codeine,[17] as well as morphine glucuronide), if present in urine in sufficient concentration, will participate in the assay in a manner indistinguishable from morphine. Either a drug or its metabolites may cross-react and it is highly desirable that the extent and significance of the cross-reactivity be determined. This is most clearly delineated by the analysis of serial samples obtained from individuals who have received the drug in question under defined circumstances (e.g., dextromethorphan[23] and poppy seeds[15]). Alternatively cross-reactivity may be determined by adding pure drug to the appropriate biological fluid and then estimating the morphine content. This procedure is less desirable since a drug may be metabolized to compounds which do not cross-react while other drugs may be metabolized to cross-reacting compounds. This may be partially overcome by testing known metabolites.

The apparent lack of specificity described above must be considered with respect to the analytical objectives. If the primary objective is to detect heroin and metabolites and not other opiates, the major cross-reactivity with codeine is clearly a disadvantage. However if the objective is to detect any opiate use the codeine cross-reactivity is advantageous. For the reasons cited above the immunoassay result should be expressed and conceptualized in units of "morphine equivalents" per ml of sample.

False-positive

This term describes the condition in which a drug is reported to be present (positive result) when in fact it is not present. A false-positive immunoassay result may be due to an error in performing the assay or reporting the result, the presence of normal biological substances in body fluids which cross-react in the assay, or the presence of cross-reacting drugs or metabolites. Since the latter two factors are in part influenced by the sensitivity, the incidence of false-positive results is partially subject to manipulation. Thus the false-positive rate may be decreased by selecting a higher concentration as the detection limits.

False-negative

This term describes the condition in which a drug is reported to be absent (negative result) when in fact it is present. While a false-negative may be due to technical error, its primary determinants are the sensitivity selected and the time course of metabolism and excretion of the drug and/or metabolites detected. It is apparent that both the incidence of false-positives and false-negatives are influenced by the degree of sensitivity selected; maximal sensitivity results in more false-positives and less false-negatives and vice versa for a decreased sensitivity level.

The second major determinant of the false-negative rate — the time course of excretion of drug — is subject to considerable variation and must be determined experimentally. Time course of excretion refers to the change in concentration of a drug or metabolite with respect to the time elapsed since the drug was administered. The time at which the sample is collected is critical as the concentration changes with time. As a generalization, body fluids obtained soon after the administration of a drug will contain higher concentrations of drug than those obtained many hours later. Exactly how much drug is present depends upon additional pharmacologic variables such as the drug and dose administered, the route of administration, the fluid examined, the state of tolerance to the drug, and the metabolism of the drug. The variation between individuals in the metabolism, distribution and excretion of drugs results in serum concentrations of some drugs which vary by a factor of 10 among patients receiving the same dose.[35] With respect to the analysis of urine, the concentration of drug is affected by still other sources of variability such as hydration, renal function and urinary pH. Thus the urinary concentration of drug is subject to wide variation and the range of values must be determined by appropriate clinical studies. This point is demonstrated by the studies of Catlin and co-workers who obtained urine from heroin addicts and determined the concentration of morphine equivalents by radioimmunoassay[23] and hemagglutination inhibition.[24] The samples obtained between 12 and 24 hr after the last use of intravenous heroin were found to contain 0.10 to 300 μg morphine equivalents/ml urine. While the majority of the samples contained 1.0 to 40.0 μg/ml the wide range of values is a reflection of the number of variables which determine the concentration of a drug in urine and illustrates the gamut of the analytical task. Clearly the detection of 300 μg/ml is quite different from detecting 0.10 μg/ml.

IMMUNOASSAY COMPARATIVE PERFORMANCE STUDIES

Factors to be considered in the selection of a diagnostic test include those described above as well as consideration of cost, analysis time, and simplicity. Within the confines of one experimental design, it is difficult if not impossible to adequately delineate each of these factors. However, there are several types of studies available which in combination permit a reasonable assessment of the current status of the immunoassays for drugs of abuse.

Elsewhere in this volume Mulé and Sunshine report their experiences with the analysis of several thousand urine samples. The data were obtained in laboratories analyzing several hundred or thousand samples per day. Accordingly, these studies are ideally designed to appraise costs, analysis time, simplicity, overall reliability, and the practical sensitivity. In addition, they provide an estimate of the percent of samples positive by these tests in the particular geographic region served by the respective laboratories. Since the studies report no clinical or pharmacological information they do not yield information relative to validity or the incidence of false-negative results, although they can relative to a reference assay.

Gorodetzky has carried out studies designed to

investigate the validity of drug detecting immuno-assays.[27,28] He defines validity as the ability of an assay to detect a drug or its metabolites in biological fluids after human drug administration.[2] Thus, validity includes sensitivity, specificity, and other pharmacologic variables discussed above. These studies, summarized elsewhere in this volume, utilized human post-addict volunteers in whom the important variables of dose, route of administration, and urine collection time intervals were carefully controlled. The extent to which these findings can be generalized to a nonconfined population of heroin addicts using unknown doses is difficult to assess. However, it should be noted that the results reported by Gorodetzky are similar to the studies reported in the subsequent paragraphs.

Our studies[23,24,30] have been directed to obtaining and analyzing samples obtained from a population of heroin addicts under circumstances which are typical of the conditions which prevail in a drug treatment clinic. The subjects were 74 males applying for admission to one of the methadone clinics maintained by the Narcotics Treatment Administration in Washington, D.C. The inherent difficulty of studying a population of out-patient heroin addicts precluded estimation of several variables. Thus, all attempts to establish the most recent dose or effect of heroin were unsuccessful. Therefore a concerted effort was directed toward defining a population according to clinical evidence of tolerance to and dependence on heroin. During the interview it was established that each had used heroin one or more times each day for at least one year and that the "dose" of heroin required to produce euphoria had increased. Dependence was established by a spontaneous history of typical abstinence symptoms when deprived of heroin for more than 12 to 24 hr. In this manner, the individuals were clinically defined as tolerant to and dependent on heroin. In addition, the time elapsed between the last use of heroin and collection was considered critical. This interval was very carefully estimated by repeated direct and indirect questions. Accordingly, the intervals obtained are considered as accurate as possible under the circumstances. The route of administration was established as intravenous both by history and the presence of needle marks adjacent to veins.

Each sample was divided into aliquots and analyzed in a blind design by each of five different methods as previously described.[30] The results for four of these methods from the analysis of one urine sample obtained from each of 74 individuals are summarized in Table 1. For all assays the percent positive decreases as a function of time elapsed and increasing sensitivity (lower detection limit). It is apparent however that at the 0.025 μg/ml sensitivity the percent positive by RIA and HI is 96 to 100 during the initial 48 hr, and subsequently declines rather precipitously. In contrast, the percent positive by FRAT and TLC falls to 78 and 35 respectively during the 13 to 24-hr interval.

To examine the question of what effect changing the sensitivity has on the percent positive the RIA and HI data are presented at four different sensitivities. This computation is possible because the data were quantitative.[31] The agreement between the percent positive by either RIA or HI at each sensitivity is close. It is apparent however that although a change in sensitivity from 0.025 to 0.10 does not significantly reduce the percent positive during the 0 to 12- or 13 to 24-hr interval, the change does result in significant reductions after 24 hr. It is concluded that for this population of addicts a sensitivity of 0.025 μg/ml is required in order to achieve a percent positive of 95 or more for 48 hr. The sensitivity could be reduced to 0.10 μg/ml and still result in greater than 90% positives. This change would be advantageous since a decrease in sensitivity generally means less false-positives and consequently greater confidence in the positive results.

GUIDELINES

Consideration of the concepts and data presented above suggests guidelines for applying the drug detecting immunoassays and for interpreting the immunoassay results. The ideal screening test for morphine should be sensitive, specific, rapid, simple to perform, inexpensive, and provide a high ratio of analyses per analyst. For most of these parameters, the immunoassays are competitive with or an improvement over the nonserologic tests. Immunoassays are particularly well suited for those laboratories analyzing hundreds of samples per day. Furthermore they can be partially automated and may provide an answer in less than 1 hr. The latter characteristic is useful for those situations where a rapid preliminary result is essential, for example, triage points or hospital

TABLE 1

The percent of urine samples positive for morphine or morphine equivalent as a function of the assay employed, the sensitivity of the assay and the hours since heroin was used. One sample was obtained from each of 74 known chronic heroin addicts.

Percent Positive

Assay	Sensitivity µg/ml	Hours Since Heroin			
		0−12 (18)[a]	13−24 (27)	25−48 (14)	49−96 (15)
RIA	0.025[e]	100	96	100	53
	0.10	100	93	57	40
	0.50	89	78	43	0
	1.00	78	70	43	0
HI	0.025[e]	100	96	100	60
	0.10	100	93	64	27
	0.50	94	85	50	13
	1.00	94	74	43	0
FRAT	0.50[e]	100	78	64	13
TLC[b]	c	87[15][d]	35[20]	50[10]	8[12]

[a]Parentheses indicate the number of individuals (and samples) obtained and analyzed during each time interval.
[b]The TLC procedure included on organic extraction but not a hydrolysis step.[36]
[c]The TLC sensitivity is estimated to be 0.50 to 1.0 g/ml.[30]
[d]Brackets indicate the number of samples analyzed by TLC, which is less than the other assays due to insufficient sample volume.
[e]Lowest recommended sensitivity.

emergency rooms. If the major program requirements are high specificity and low volume, such as the forensic laboratory, the immunoassay is not the method of choice.

The negative immunoassay result is very strong evidence that the drug in question is not present in excess of the sensitivity utilized. Accordingly, these samples require no further analysis. The positive result is evidence that the drug is present and the greater the quantity reported the stronger the evidence. Cross-reactions do occur, and therefore, for the purpose of definitive identification it is essential that the result be confirmed by a second and nonserological method. Thus, the immunoassay is not well suited for situations in which the positive rate is high and many samples will require confirmation.

Individuals interpreting the results of immunoassays should be aware of the interrelationships between sensitivity, specificity, time since drug use, and false-positive and false-negative rates. Periodic comparisons of the results with the

clinical information obtained from the patients are essential. Sensitivity should be selected to yield a positive result in more than 90% of samples obtained within 24 hr of the last drug use provided that this sensitivity does not result in an intolerable false-positive rate. Failure to meet this specification has differing implications depending on the clinical setting. For the drug treatment clinic it will result in an underestimation of the extent of continuing heroin abuse in abstinant or methadone maintained patients, and impair the ability to support the diagnosis of chronic heroin addiction with a positive sample. For screening populations with a low rate of heroin use, insufficient 24-hr sensitivity may result in the failure to detect those few individuals who are using heroin and for whom early therapeutic intervention may be beneficial.

SUMMARY

Definitions are presented for terms frequently

used with respect to the immunoassays designed to detect drugs of abuse. The definitions are useful for the discussion of studies designed to compare and evaluate the immunoassays. The experimental design of these studies are elaborated in order to emphasize the desirability of correlating clinical information with test results. In this fashion, the critical and inextricable interrelationships between sensitivity, specificity, and time course of detection are demonstrated. In turn, this information suggests the proper applications of immunoassays and interpretation of the assay results.

ACKNOWLEDGMENT

The expert assistance of Ms. Kathleen Ellsworth in the preparation of the manuscript is gratefully acknowledged.

This work was supported in part by a research grant from SAODAP (HSM-401378) and NIMH (DA00653).

REFERENCES

1. **Way, E. L. and Adler, T. K.,** The biological disposition of morphine and its surrogates, *Bull. W.H.O.,* 25, 227, 1961.
2. **Gorodetzky, C. W.,** Urinalysis: Practical and Theoretical Considerations, Proceedings of the Fourth National Conference on Methadone Treatment, 1972, 155.
3. **Mulé, S. J.,** Identification of narcotics, barbiturates, amphetamines, tranquilizers, and psychotomimetics in human urine, *J. Chromatogr.,* 39, 302, 1969.
4. **Mulé, S. J.,** Methods for the analysis of narcotic analgesics and amphetamines, *J. Chromatogr. Sci.,* 10, 275, 1972.
5. **Dole, V. P., Crowther, A., Johnson, J., Montsalvatge, M., Biller, B., and Nelson, S. S.,** Detention of narcotic, sedative and amphetamine drugs in urine, *N.Y. State J. Med.,* 471, 1972.
6. **Mulé, S. J. and Hushin, P. L.,** Semiautomated fluorometric assay for submicrogram quantities of morphine and quinine in human biological material, *Anal. Chem.,* 43, 708, 1971.
7. **Kaistha, K. K. and Jaffe, J. H.,** TLC techniques for identification of narcotics, barbiturates, and CNS stimulants in a drug abuse urine screening program, *J. Pharm. Sci.,* 61, 679, 1972.
8. **Kaistha, K. K.,** Drug abuse screening programs: Detection procedures, development costs, street-sample analysis, and field tests, *J. Pharm. Sci.,* 61, 655, 1972.
9. **Finkle, B. S.,** Forensic toxicology of drug abuse: A status report, *Anal. Chem.,* 9, 19, 1972.
10. **Dole, V. P., Kim, W. K., and Eglitis, I.,** Detection of narcotic drugs, tranquilizers, amphetamines, and barbiturates in urine, *J.A.M.A.,* 198, 349, 1966.
11. **Mulé, S. J., Bastos, M. L., Jukofsky, D., and Safer, E.,** Routine identification of drugs of abuse in human urine. II Development and application of the XAD-2 resin column method, *J. Chromatogr.,* 63, 289, 1971.
12. **Bastos, M. L., Jukofsky, D., Saffer, E., Chedikel, M., and Mulé, S. J.,** Modifications of the XAD-2 resin column method for the extraction of drugs of abuse from human urine, *J. Chromatogr.,* 71, 549, 1972.
13. **Sansur, M., Buccafuri, A., and Morgenstern, S.,** Automated fluorometric method for the determination of morphine in urine, *J. Assoc. Off. Anal. Chem.,* 55, 880, 1972.
14. **Spector, S.,** Quantitative determination of morphine in serum by radioimmunoassay, *J. Pharmacol. Exp. Ther.,* 178, 253, 1971.
15. **Adler, F. L., Liu, C. T., and Catlin, D. H.,** Immunological studies on heroin addiction I. Methodology and application of a hemagglutination-inhibition test for detection of morphine, *Clin. Immunol. Immunopathol.,* 1, 53, 1972.
16. **Rubenstein, K. E., Schneider, R. J., and Ullman, E. F.,** 'Homogeneous' enzyme immunoassay. A new immunochemical technique, *Biochem. Biophys. Res. Comm.,* 47, 846, 1972.
17. **Leute, R. K., Ullman, E.F., and Goldstein, A.,** Spin immunoassay of opiate narcotics in urine and saliva, *J.A.M.A.,* 211, 1231, 1972.
18. **Leute, R. K., Ullman, E. F., Goldstein, A., and Herzenberg, L. A.,** Spin immunoassay technique for determination of morphine, *Nature, New Biol.,* 236, 93, 1972.
19. **Liu, C. T. and Adler, F. L.,** Immunological studies on drug addiction I. Antibodies reactive with methadone and their use for detection of the drug, *J. Immunol.,* 1973, in press.
20. **Flynn, E. J. and Spector, S.,** Determination of barbiturate derivatives by radioimmunoassay, *J. Pharm. Exp. Ther.,* 181, 547, 1972.
21. **Adler, F. L. and Liu, C. T.,** Detection of morphine by hemagglutination inhibition, *J. Immunol.,* 106, 1684, 1971.
22. **Spector, S. and Parker, C. W.,** Morphine: Radioimmunoassay, *Science,* 168, 3247, 1970.
23. **Catlin, D. H., Cleeland, R., and Grunberg, E.,** A sensitive rapid radioimmunoassay for morphine and immunologically related substances in urine and serum, *Clin. Chem.,* 19, 216, 1973.

24. Catlin, D. H., Adler, F. J., and Liu, C. T., Immunological studies on heroin addiction II. Applications of a sensitive hemagglutination-inhibition test for detecting morphine to diagnostic problems in chronic heroin addiction, *Clin. Immunol. Immunopathol.*, 1, 446, 1973.

25. Bastiani, R. J., Phillips, R. C., Schneider, R. S., and Ullman, E. F., Homogeneous immunochemical drug assays, *Am. J. Med. Technol.*, 39, 211, 1973.

26. Mulé, S. J., Urinalysis of 39,350 samples for drugs subject to abuse in a methadone maintenance treatment program, *Br. J. Addict.*, in press, 1973.

27. Gorodetzky, C. W., Time course of morphine (M) detection in human urine after iv heroin (H), *Fed. Proc.*, 31, 528 Abs., 1972.

28. Gorodetzky, C. W., Time course of morphine (M) detection in human urine after IV morphine, *Fed. Proc.*, 32, 764 Abs., 1973.

29. Gorodetzky, C. W., Sensitivity of thin-layer chromatography for detection of opiods, cocaine and quinine, *Toxicol. Appl. Pharmacol.*, 23, 611, 1971.

30. Catlin, D. H., Urine testing: A comparison of five different methods for detecting morphine, *Am. J. Clin. Pathol.*, in press, 1973.

31. Mulé, S. J., Detection and identification of drugs of dependence, in *Clinical and Biological Aspects of Drug Dependence,* Mulé, S. J. and Brill, H., Eds., CRC Press, Cleveland, 1972.

32. Spector, S. and Flynn, E. J., Barbiturates: Radioimmunoassay, *Science,* 174, 1036, 1971.

33. Schnoll, S. H., Vogel, W. H., and Odstrchel, G., The specificity of anti-mescaline antibody produced in rabbits, *Fed. Proc. Abstr.,* 33, 719, 1973.

34. Williams, T. A. and Pittman, K. A., A radioimmunoassay for pentozacine, *Fed. Proc.,* 33, 719 Abs., 1973.

35. Koch-Weser, J., Serum drug concentrations as therapeutic guides, *N. Engl. J. Med.,* 287, 227, 1972.

36. Davidow, B., Li Petri, N., and Quame, B., A thin-layer chromatographic screening procedure for detecting drug abuse, *Am. J. Clin. Pathol.,* 50, 714, 1968.

A COMPARISON OF IMMUNOASSAY METHODS FOR THE DETECTION OF DRUGS SUBJECT TO ABUSE*

S. J. Mulé and M. L. Bastos

TABLE OF CONTENTS

INTRODUCTION

An increase in the number of programs for the treatment of drug dependence as well as current federal regulations have created the need for rapid, sensitive, reliable, and inexpensive methods for the detection and identification of drugs subject to abuse. In order to meet this challenge, immuno-chemical techniques have been applied to the detection of drugs in biological materials. Four methods were recently developed and are currently available. These are (1) radioimmuno-assay (RIA); (2) free radical assay technique (FRAT); (3) enzyme multiplied immunoassay technique (EMIT); and (4) hemagglutination in-hibition (HI).

It is the purpose of this communication to compare the immunoassays (except FRAT) for drugs subject to abuse with each other, and with thin-layer chromatographic and fluorometric methods. The major emphasis will be upon the reliability and/or validity of the new technology.

MATERIALS AND METHODS

The urines were analyzed by thin-layer chroma-tography,[1-4] radioimmunoassay,[5,6] enzyme multiplied immunoassay technique,[7,8] hemag-glutination inhibition,[9,10] and spectrophoto-fluorometry.[11,12] All chemicals were of reagent grade.

RESULTS

Comparison data for the detection of morphine in 422 human urine samples appear in Table 1. Using thin-layer chromatography (TLC), 94.3% of the samples were negative and 5.7% of the samples were positive. The number of positive samples increased to 13.7, 14.0, and 25.5% with the EMIT, HI, and RIA assays, respectively. The positive detection level used for these three assays (low sensitivity) was 0.5 $\mu g/ml$ of morphine. An in-crease in the sensitivity level to 30 ng/ml of morphine (high sensitivity) increased the number

*This work was supported in part by U.S. Public Health Service Grant DA-00061-03.

TABLE 1

A Percentage Comparison of Urine Screening Methods for the Detection of Morphine in 422 Human Urine Samples

Results	TLC[a]	Low sensitivity[b] (0.5 µg/ml and above)			High sensitivity[c] (30 ng/ml and above)		Quinine[d] Indirect technique (ATS) (0.1 µg/ml and above)
		EMIT	HI	RIA	HI	RIA	
True negative (confirmed by TLC)	94.3	86.3	86.0	74.5	67.3	63.6	70.0
Positive	5.7	13.7	14.0	25.5	32.7	36.4	30.0
True positives (confirmed by TLC)	–	5.0	5.0	5.7	4.7	5.7	5.0
False positives[e] (unconfirmed by TLC)	–	8.7	9.0	19.8	28.0	30.7	25.0
False negatives[e] (unconfirmed by TLC)	–	0.5	0.7	0.0	1.0	0.0	1.3

[a]TLC, thin-layer chromatography of the urine samples using methods and techniques reported previously (Mulé et al., *J. Chromatogr.*, 63, 289, 1971; Bastos, M. L. et al., *J. Chromatogr.*, 71, 549, 1971).

[b]EMIT, enzyme multiplied immunoassay technique (opiate assay); HI, hemagglutination inhibition; RIA, radio-immunoassay technique. Results obtained using a maximal sensitivity level of 0.5 µg/ml of drug.

[c]Results obtained using a maximal sensitivity level of 30 ng/ml of morphine.

[d]Determined by the automated turret spectrofluorometric (ATS) method (Mulé and Hushin, *Anal. Chem.*, 43, 708, 1971). Maximal sensitivity at 0.1 µg/ml of quinine. The presence of quinine is indicative of heroin usage. The samples subsequently were acid hydrolyzed and subjected to thin-layer chromatography (Mulé et al., *J. Chromatogr.*, 55, 255, 1971).

[e]False positives and negatives as compared to thin-layer chromatography (TLC). The maximal detection level for morphine by the TLC techniques utilized was 1 µg/ml.

of positive samples for the HI and RIA assays to 32.7 and 36.4%, respectively. Therefore, it is quite evident that a sample is negative only within the definition of the sensitivity of the analysis. In the case of the automated turret spectrophotofluorometric (ATS) method, the percentage of positive samples also includes those suspicious for quinine. Therefore, a fraction of the samples positive by the immunoassay methods and the ATS technique were confirmed by TLC (4.7 to 5.7%). This does not imply that all the unconfirmed TLC positives (8.7 to 30.7%) were false. The maximal practical level of sensitivity for TLC is about 1 to 2 µg/ml of morphine and therefore, a fair percentage of the unconfirmed by TLC (false-positive) were simply due to the lower sensitivity limits of TLC in comparison to the immunoassay methods. This fact is even more obvious with the high-sensitivity data where the unconfirmed by TLC (false-positives) were 28.0 and 30.7% for HI and RIA, respectively. Primarily due to the 0.1 µg/ml detection level with the ATS technique, a high incidence of unconfirmed positives by TLC (25.0%) was observed. The negatives unconfirmed by TLC (false-negative) were in all cases quite small, ranging from 0.0 to 1.3%. Thus, the false

negative percentage with the immunoassay techniques appears to be one percent or less as compared to TLC.

The data on cross-reactivity of the various immunoassays as well as the fluorometric technique for narcotic agonists and antagonists appear in Table 2. In the RIA test, only codeine was apparently more sensitive to this assay than morphine. Drugs such as heroin, dihydromorphinone, levorphanol, and dihydromorphine were detected almost as readily as morphine. There was a very low level of cross-reactivity for naloxone, pseudomorphine, apomorphine, *d*-and *l*-methorphan, methadone, *d*-propoxyphene, and cyclazocine.

In the HI assay, dihydromorphine, dihydromorphinone, codeine, and heroin demonstrated a high degree of cross-reactivity, whereas normorphine, nalorphine, levorphanol, *d*- and *l*-methorphan as well as *d*-propoxyphene provided a very small degree of cross-reactivity.

The EMIT assay for opiates included several drugs with a low level of cross-reactivity, i.e., *d*-and *l*-methorphan, normorphine, and nalorphine. Codeine was the only drug that was more reactive in this assay than morphine. It was also possible to

TABLE 2

Concentration of Drugs in Urine Which Cross-react When Submitted to the Same Screening Procedure. Values Equivalent to 0.5 μg/ml of Morphine

Drug	Immunoassays						Fluorometry[b]
	RIA	R.R.[c]	HI	R.R.	EMIT[a]	R.R.	R.R.
Normorphine	20.8	(0.024)	100.0	(0.005)	22.2	(0.023)	15.5 (0.032)
Codeine	0.38	(1.316)	0.50	(1.000)	0.39	(1.282)	N.R.[f]
Diacetylmorphine (Heroin)	0.50	(1.000)	1.20	(0.416)	1.2	(0.417)	10.2 (0.049)
N-Allylnormorphine (Nalorphine)	5.0	(0.100)	200.0	(0.003)	7.9	(0.063)	1.2 (0.417)
N-Allyl,7,8,dihydro-14-hydroxy-normorphinone (Naloxone)	145.0	(0.003)			N.R.		N.R.
Dihydromorphinone (Dilaudid)	0.60	(0.833)	1.50	(0.333)	1.3	(0.385)	N.R.
Dihydromorphine	0.75	(0.667)	0.75	(0.667)	1.9	(0.263)	0.40 (1.250)
Pseudomorphine	145.0	(0.003)			N.R.		
Apomorphine	175.0	(0.003)			N.R.		
Morphine glucuronide					1.3	(0.385)	N.R.
1-3-Hydroxy-N-methylmorphinan (Levorphanol)	1.0	(0.500)	25.0	(0.020)	3.1	(0.161)	N.R.
d-3-Methoxy-N-methylmorphinan[d] (Dextromethorphan)	439.4	(0.001)	N.R.		134.0	(0.004)	
1-3-Methoxy-N-methylmorphinan (Levomethorphan)	115	(0.004)	400.0	(0.001)	50.0	(0.010)	
2-Ethylidene-1,5-dimethyl-3,3-diphenylpyrrolidine					N.R.		
2-Ethyl-5-methyl-3,3-diphenyl-1-pyrroline					500	(0.001)	
Methadone	890.0	(0.001)	N.R.		N.R.		
d-Propoxyphene (Darvon)[e]	340.0	(0.001)	50.0	(0.010)	N.R.		
Cyclazocine	190.0	(0.003)			N.R.		N.R.

[a]EMIT = assay for opiates.

[b]Technicon autoanalyzer technique as described by Sansur et al., *J. Assoc. Offic. Anal. Chem.*, 55, 880, 1972.

[c]R.R. = Relative reactivity in comparison to 0.5 μg/ml of morphine.

[d]Among 5 urine samples positive for dextromethorphan by TLC on routine urine screening, 2 were negative with RIA, HI, and EMIT; 2 were positive with RIA, HI, and EMIT (RIA for morphine about 600 ng/ml) and 1 was positive with RIA (RIA for morphine about 250 ng/ml) and HI, but negative with EMIT. No sample had morphine and one had quinine.

[e]Among 4 urine samples with positive TLC result for d-propoxyphene, two were negative by the immunoassays for morphine, 1 was positive with RIA (RIA for morphine about 210 ng/ml) and the other was positive with RIA (RIA for morphine about 600 ng/ml), HI and EMIT. No sample had morphine or quinine present.

[f]N.R. refers to no reaction at a concentration of 500 μg/ml and in the fluorometric assay 10 mg/ml.

detect morphine glucuronide at a ratio of about 3:1 in comparison to morphine (R.R. = 0.385).

The Technicon® autoanalyzer was used to determine the cross-reactivity of several narcotic drugs by the spectrofluorometric technique. Of the drugs tested, only dihydromorphine appeared as easily detected as morphine (1:1 ratio, RR = 1.25). The other drugs (normorphine, heroin, and nalorphine) were detected at levels of 2.4 to 31 times the concentration of morphine and many structurally related drugs (naloxone, dihydromorphinone, levorphanol, and morphine glucuronide) were not detected by this technique.

The relative reactivity data provide a direct comparison on a ratio basis of all the drugs (Table 2) in comparison to 0.5 μg/ml of morphine equivalency for each assay.

A summary of the validity (reliability) of various EMIT assays as compared to thin-layer chromatography is provided in Table 3. A total of true results for all the assays ranged from 87 to 95%. The percentage of false positives varied from 2.6 to 12.5%. The percentage of false-negatives ranged from 0 to 2.3%. The total unconfirmed percentage of these assays (false-negative and false-positive) was 5 to 13%. It is obvious that the false negative figures for these assays in comparison to TLC were insignificant. The percentage of

TABLE 3

Comparison of the EMIT Assays With Thin-layer Chromatography[a] in Human Urine Samples for Drugs Subject to Abuse

	EMIT assays[b]									
	Methadone		Opiate		Amphetamine		Barbiturate		Cocaine[d]	
Results	N[c]	%	N	%	N	%	N	%	N	%
True positive[e]	3,412	42.7	77	1.6	8	1.1	20	3.2	50	64.9
True negative[e]	4,194	52.4	4,584	92.8	651	85.7	609	91.7	18	23.4
Total	7,606	95.1	4,661	94.4	659	86.8	629	94.7	68	88.3
False positive[f]	206	2.6	275	5.6	95	12.5	34	5.1	9	11.7
False negative[f]	187	2.3	4	0.1	5	0.7	1	0.2	0	0.0
Total	393	4.9	279	5.7	100	13.2	35	5.3	9	11.7

[a]Thin-layer chromatography performed as described in Table 1.
[b]EMIT assays performed as described under methods.
[c]N = the number of samples.
[d]All samples analyzed were confirmed by the butylated ecgonine method of M. Bastos, D. Jukofsky, and S. J. Mulé (manuscript in preparation).
[e]Confirmed by thin-layer chromatography.
[f]Unconfirmed by thin-layer chromatography. Further analysis of the cocaine data indicated that all false positive samples (9) were at concentrations below 3 μg/ml of benzoylecgonine and thus below the maximal sensitivity of the TLC method for confirmation.

false positives was certainly significant with the opiate, amphetamine, barbiturate, and cocaine assays. In the case of cocaine, it was subsequently shown that all the false positive samples were due to the lower sensitivity level of the thin-layer chromtographic technique[13] for butylated ecgonine (3 to 5 μg/ml).

All the samples proven positive by EMIT and negative by TLC contained benzoylecgonine concentrations of 3 or less μg/ml. A difference in sensitivity between the EMIT amphetamine assay (2.0 μg/ml) and TLC (5 μg/ml) also contributed to the false positive percentage of 12.5. The false-positive values for the methadone, opiate, and barbiturate assays were not as apparent, possibly due to some extent to the low sensitivity of TLC in comparison to EMIT. The maximal practical level of detection for our TLC techniques was 1 to 5 μg/ml for these drugs in comparison to 0.5 to 2.0 μg/ml for the EMIT assays.

Tables 4, 5, and 6 summarize the data concerning cross-reactivity of related compounds in the amphetamine, methadone, and barbiturate EMIT assays. The tables are self-explanatory. However, it is noteworthy to mention that two of the primary metabolites (cyclized) of methadone did not appear to interfere in the methadone EMIT assay.

A comparison of the morphine confirmation

TABLE 4

Cross-reactivity of Amphetamine and Related Compounds in the EMIT Amphetamine Assay[a]

Compound	Equivalent to 1 μg/ml of amphetamine	Relative reactivity
Amphetamine	1.0	1.00
Phenethylamine	3.1	0.32
Phenylpropanolamine	5.0	0.20
Methamphetamine	0.92	1.08
Methylphenidate	>50	>0.02
Phenmetrazine	0.95	1.05
Mephentermine	1.6	0.62
Phentermine	1.6	0.62
Benzphetamine	3.0	0.33
Cyclopentamine	3.0	0.33
Ephedrine	4.5	0.22
Nylidrin	3.7	0.27
Isoxsuprine	5.0	0.20
Methoxyphenamine	3.0	0.33
p-Hydroxyamphetamine	80	0.02
Tyramine	∞	—
Tyrosine	∞	—
Phenylephrine	107	0.01
Isoproterenol	∞	—
Methylhexamine	10	0.10
Pheniramine	102	0.01
Phenylalanine	∞	—

[a]Portions of the data were kindly provided by Dr. R. J. Bastiani of the Syva Corporation, Palo Alto, California.

TABLE 5

Cross-reactivity of Methadone, Methadone Metabolites, and Other Narcotic Drugs in the Methadone EMIT Assay

Compound	Equivalent to 0.5 μg/ml of methadone	Relative reactivity
Methadone	0.5	1.00
Meperidine	500	0.001
2-Ethylidene-1,5-dimethyl-3,3-Diphenylpyrrolidine	NR[a]	–
2-Ethyl-5-methyl-3,3-diphenyl-1-pyrroline	NR	–
d-Propoxyphene	NR	–

[a]NR = no cross-reactivity at a maximum concentration of 500 μg/ml.

TABLE 6

Cross-reactivity of Barbiturates in the EMIT Barbiturate Assay[a]

Drug	Equivalent to 1 μg/ml of secobarbital	Relative reactivity
Secobarbital	1.0	1.0
Phenobarbital	2.0	0.50
Pentobarbital	1.1	0.90
Amobarbital	1.8	0.55
Butabarbital	5.4	0.18
Heptabarbital	2.4	0.42
Mephobarbital	0.3	3.33
Thiamylal	0.6	1.66
Talbutal	1.8	0.55
Thiopental	0.7	1.42
Aprobarbital	11.5	0.08
Metharbital	75.0	0.01
Barbital	60.0	0.02
Probarbital	30.0	0.03
Glutethimide[b]	50.0	0.02

[a]The data were kindly provided by Dr. R. J. Bastiani of the Syva Corporation, Palo Alto, California.
[b]Nonbarbiturate sedative.

rate from methadone positive and negative human urines is presented in Table 7. The number of EMIT positive results between the two groups was not statistically significant. However, the morphine confirmation rate for the methadone-positive samples was 12.8% in comparison to 26.9% for the morphine-negative samples ($P < 0.001$). The false-positive rate was 73.1% and 87.2% for the negative and positive methadone

urine samples, respectively. This clearly indicates that methadone, its metabolites, or unknown biochemical factors contribute to a low morphine confirmation rate in methadone-positive urine samples. The cyclized pyrroline methadone metabolite provided a ratio of 1,000:1 (RR = 0.001) in comparison to morphine in the opiate assay and the pyrrolidine metabolite did not react at a maximum concentration of 500 μg/ml.

The advantages and disadvantages of the various immunoassays are outlined in Table 8. In essence, the major considerations were sensitivity, specificity, validity or reliability, technical simplicity, and, of course, cost. An evaluation of the primary purpose of the program must also be considered before final decision is made concerning any analytical technique to be used for the detection of psychoactive drugs.

DISCUSSION

In this communication, an attempt was made to compare three immunoassay techniques (RIA, HI, and EMIT) and fluorometric methods with thin-layer chromatography. Primary emphasis was placed upon sensitivity, specificity (cross-reactivity), and reliability of the immunoassays to detect drugs subject to abuse.

The immunoassays unquestionably were more sensitive in detecting drugs than thin-layer chromatographic techniques. The maximal practical levels of detection using TLC ranged from 1 to 5 μg/ml for the opiates, barbiturates, and amphetamine group of drugs. The sensitivity values for the immunoassays ranged from 30 ng/ml of morphine for HI to 500 ng/ml of morphine for EMIT. RIA reliably provided sensitivity values of 60 ng/ml for morphine and a concentration of 200 to 300 ng/ml was detectable for morphine (100 ng/ml for quinine) with the fluorometric techniques (ATS and Technicon). A high percentage of positive urines unconfirmed by TLC (8 to 32%) may have been truly positive but were present at concentrations undetectable by TLC. This certainly was the situation with cocaine and may well have been the case with other drugs in some instances.

The percentage of false-negatives for all the immunoassays tested was quite low (usually 1% or less). This of course adds further evidence to the reliability of these assays as an exclusion test for drugs subject to abuse.

Lack of specificity (cross-reactivity) was com-

TABLE 7

Comparison of the Morphine Confirmation Rate from Methadone Positive and Negative Human Urine Samples

	Methadone Negative	%	Methadone Positive	%	P-Value
N[a]	10,479		7,404		
EMIT positive[b]	867	8.3	563	7.6	NS
Morphine confirmation rate[c] (confirmed by TLC)	233	26.9	72	12.8	P < 0.001 (Z = 6.35)
False positive rate	634	73.1	491	87.2	

[a]N = Number of urine samples analyzed.
[b]EMIT assay for opiates as described under methods.
[c]Urines subjected to acid hydrolysis prior to extraction and TLC.

TABLE 8

Comparison of Screening Methods for Morphine

	Advantages	Disadvantages
EMIT	(1) Immediate results, very convenient for screening purposes (2) Results obtained objectively (direct printout) (3) Quantitative evaluation in the range 0.5 to about 5 µg/ml (4) Fair degree of specificity (5) Detects morphine glucuronide (6) Available for opiates, barbiturates, amphetamines, methadone and cocaine	(1) Some false positive results observed in urine with high blank values (normal lysozyme activity) (2) pH may be critical when handling aged samples (3) Sensitivity not quite as good as other immunoassay techniques (4) Requires instrumentation (5) High price of reagents
HI	(1) Low price, no equipment, simple technique (2) Maximum sensitivity (3 to 30 ng/ml) (3) Flexibility for screening at different sensitivity levels (4) Detects morphine glucuronide	(1) Time delay between test and results, which may be troublesome on large scale screening (90-min incubation) (2) Subjective reading or interpretation of results (3) Urine sediment may cause trouble in interpreting the results (4) Available at present only for opiates (5) Poor quality control on currently available reagents
RIA	(1) Quantitative evaluation in the range 30 to 60 ng/ml (dilutions may extend the range) (2) Maximum sensitivity (60 ng/ml) (3) Results obtained objectively (4) Fair degree of specificity (5) Detects morphine glucuronide	(1) Time delay between test and final estimation of results (2) Technical skills required for handling radioactive materials (3) High price of reagents and instrumentation (4) Large number of false positives when a 60 ng/ml sensitivity level is used as a limiting value (confirmed by TLC) (5) Available at present only for opiates

mon to all the immunoassays and varied from values greater than 1 to less than 0.001 (relative-reactivity). In almost all cases, the values for drugs other than morphine in the immunoassays were less reactive, except for codeine which was more sensitive, i.e., 380 ng/ml (RR = 1.32) in comparison to 500 ng/ml of morphine (RIA). Of the drugs tested with the Technicon fluorometric method, only dihydromorphine was apparently equal in sensitivity to morphine. Most of the drugs did not react or were less sensitive than morphine. The ATS fluorometric technique[11] was capable of detecting normorphine and nalorphine almost as well as morphine. Non-narcotic drugs apparently did not react fluorometrically.[11,12]

All the EMIT assays developed were tested and compared to TLC for reliability. The total false percentage ranged from 5 to 13% whereas the total true confirmed percentage ranged from 87 to 95%. Other than sensitivity factors, some of the unconfirmed positives might be due to native lysozyme activity in the urine as well as unknown biochemical and nutritional factors and possibly unidentified drugs and/or metabolites.

All the EMIT assays demonstrated a fair degree of cross-reactivity (nonspecificity) although in most cases the individual assay was most sensitive for the parent compound in the assay. In view of these facts, it is evident that an additional analysis must be conducted in order to confirm the presence of any drug when using the EMIT system to screen for drugs of abuse. *In fact, confirmation methods are required regardless of the immunoassay method used to detect or screen for psychoactive drugs.*

A rather interesting fact was observed in the EMIT opiate assay when methadone-positive urines were compared with urines free of methadone. The rate of confirmation for morphine in the latter case was twice as great as that obtained with the methadone-positive urines. This clearly indicated that methadone in high concentrations ($>$ than 500 μg/ml) or metabolites might directly interfere in the EMIT assay to increase the false-positive rate. In the case of the cyclized methadone metabolites, there appears to be cross-reactivity at 500 μg/ml for pyrroline and no reaction with the pyrrolidine metabolite through 500 μg/ml. Of course, other drugs and metabolites of methadone,[14] as well as nutritional and biochemical factors, may play a role in the false-positive rate observed with the methadone-positive urines.

The major advantage of the immunoassay technique is sensitivity as compared to other methods. The major disadvantage is cross-reactivity or lack of specificity. Factors such as cost of the analysis (reagents and instrumentation) as well as the technical skills needed to conduct the assays and the time required to perform a test are important but secondary to sensitivity and specificity.

The immunoassays are reliable and valid within the context of the inherent limitations described. Thus, these tests lend themselves quite readily to urine screening programs and are fully reliable as an exclusion test for drug usage. However, all positive results require confirmation by additional analyses other than an immunossay test, as stated previously.

ACKNOWLEDGMENT

The authors are grateful to Dr. R. J. Bastiani for the data provided, to Dr. F. Adler for the HI reagents, and to D. Jukofsky and M. Chedekel for excellent technical assistance.

REFERENCES

1. **Mulé, S. J.,** Routine identification of drugs of abuse in human urine 1. Application of fluorometry, thin-layer and gas-liquid chromatography, *J. Chromatogr.,* 55, 255, 1971.
2. **Mulé, S. J., Bastos, M. L., Jukofsky, D., and Saffer, E.,** Routine identification of drugs of abuse in human urine II. Development and application of the XAD-2 resin column method, *J. Chromatogr.,* 63, 289, 1971.
3. **Bastos, M. L., Jukofsky, D., Saffer, E., Chedekel, M., and Mulé, S. J.,** Modifications of the XAD-2 resin column method for the extraction of drugs of abuse from human urine, *J. Chromatogr.,* 71, 549, 1972.
4. **Bastos, M. L., Jukofsky, D. and Mulé, S. J.,** Routine identification of drugs of abuse in human urine, III. Differential elution of the XAD-2 resin, *J. Chromatogr.,* in press.
5. **Spector, S. and Parker, C. W.,** Morphine: Radioimmunoassay, *Science,* 168, 1347, 1970.
6. **Spector, S.,** Quantitative determination of morphine in serum by radioimmunoassay, *J. Pharmacol. Exp. Ther.,* 178, 253, 1971.
7. **Rubenstein, K. E., Schneider, R. S., and Ullman, E. F.,** "Homogenous" enzyme immunoassay, a new immunochemical technique, *Biochem. Biophys. Res. Commun.,* 47, 846, 1972.
8. *Emit^{TM} Operators Manual,* Syva Corporation, Palo Alto, California, October, 1972.
9. **Adler, F. and Liu, Chi-tan,** Detection of morphine by hemagglutination-inhibition, *J. Immunol.,* 106, 1684, 1971.

10. **Adler, F., Liu, Chi-tan, and Catlin, D. H.,** Immunological studies on heroin addiction. 1. Methodology and application of a hemagglutination inhibition test for detection of morphine, *Clin. Immunol. Immunopathol.,* 1, 53, 1972.

11. **Mule, S. J. and Hushin, P. L.,** Semiautomated assay for submicrogram quantities of morphine and quinine in human biological material, *Anal. Chem.,* 43, 708, 1971.

12. **Sansur, M., Buccafurim, A., and Morgenstern, S.,** Automated fluorometric method for the determination of morphine in urine, *J. Assoc. Offic. Anal. Chem.,* 55, 880, 1972.

13. **Bastos, M. L., Jukofsky, D., and Mule, S. J.,** Detection of ecgonine in human urine: a cocaine metabolite, manuscript in preparation.

14. **Misra, A. L., Mule, S. J., Bloch, R., and Vadlamani, N. L.,** Physiologic disposition and metabolism of *levo*-methadone-1-^{3}H in nontolerant and tolerant rats, *J. Pharmacol. Exp. Ther.,* 185, 287, 1973.

A COMPARISON OF AVAILABLE IMMUNOASSAYS FOR DRUGS OF ABUSE IN URINE

W. J. Brattin and I. Sunshine

TABLE OF CONTENTS

INTRODUCTION

Immunoassay is a powerful analytical technique which has recently become available for the detection of drugs of abuse in urine. The following data have been collected in order to compare the features of the four commercially manufactured drug immunoassays, and to evaluate their proper role in the detection of drugs. The data compare the sensitivity, accuracy, precision, reliability, specificity, time, and cost of these procedures. This information has been abstracted from an on-going evaluation of many methods for the detection of drugs of abuse with the hope that this preliminary report will be helpful and timely.

MATERIAL AND METHODS

Reagents and materials required for each of the immunoassays were supplied by the manufacturers. Urine samples were obtained from patients in local methadone treatment centers. Urines of this type ("methadone urines"), which were found to be free of drugs of abuse (other than methadone) by thin-layer chromatography

(TLC), enzyme multiplied immunoassay technique (EMIT®), radioimmunoassay (RIA), and gas-liquid chromatography (GLC), were pooled and used to prepare standard solutions of the various drugs used in this study. All the drugs used were commercially available.

The procedures used for each immunoassay were those suggested by the manufacturers. For the RIA, the tritium-labeled morphine (rather than iodine-125-labeled) was used.* When samples with morphine concentrations greater than 100 ng/ml were encountered they were diluted with 0.05 M potassium phosphate pH 7 to yield final concentrations between 10 and 100 ng/ml. In the case of the hemagglutination inhibition (HI) assay, the antibody was obtained in concentrated form and was diluted each day to yield a sensitivity of 200 ng morphine/ml. All free radical assay technique (FRAT) analyses were performed by United Medical Laboratories, Portland, Oregon.†

Gas chromatography of barbiturates was by the procedure of Kananen et al. Gas chromatography of amphetamine and methadone was by the procedure of Aggarwal et al.[2] Urine (10 ml) was saturated with solid K_2CO_3/NaHCO$_3$ (1/3, w/w) buffer and extracted with 100 μl of chloroform – isopropanol (3:1 v/v). A portion of the extract (about 40 μl) was evaporated to dryness in an aluminum capsule and 2 μl of acetic anhydride were added. The capsule was sealed and subsequently analyzed on a Perkin-Elmer Model 900 gas chromatograph equipped with an automated sample injection system. The column used was 3' x 1/4" O.D. glass, packed with 3% OV-17 on 80 to 100 mesh Chromasorb W. The analysis was programmed from 130 to 280° at the rate of 12°/min. Thin-layer chromatography of cocaine and its metabolites was performed by using the general TLC procedure developed by Davidow[3] for drugs of abuse.

RESULTS:
COMPARISON OF THE IMMUNOASSAYS

While each of the four commercially available immunoassays (RIA, EMIT, FRAT, and HI) may potentially be applied to any and all drugs of abuse, morphine is the only drug for which

reagents are currently available for all four methods. Thus, morphine served as the basis of a comparison of these four techniques.

Sensitivity

For the purposes of this report, the "sensitivity" of a method is defined as the lowest concentration of morphine tested that produced a response which was distinguishable from the background response at least 90% of the time. For quantitative methods (RIA, FRAT, and EMIT) this corresponds to the concentration at which the average response minus two standard deviations is greater than the average response of the background plus two standard deviations. For HI, which was used as a qualitative method, this corresponds to the concentration at which a minimum of 90% of the samples were judged to be positive.

The sensitivity of each of the four immunoassays was evaluated by assaying a number of samples ("proficiency standards") whose concentrations were known. These were prepared by dividing a large pool of "methadone urine" into six portions and adding morphine sulfate to yield six different concentrations (0, 100, 200, 400, 600, and 1,000 ng/ml). Ten aliquots of these six solutions were withdrawn and analyzed in random order (in a "blind" fashion) by each technique. The average responses and standard deviations of each method to these samples are presented in Table 1. Based on the definition of sensitivity given above, the sensitivity of RIA is seen to be 100 ng/ml. However, since all samples were diluted 1/10 prior to assay, the actual sensitivity is 10 ng/ml. The sensitivity of FRAT is 100 ng/ml, and of EMIT is 400 ng/ml. The sensitivity of HI is adjustable, depending on the titer of the antiserum used. In this case, the sensitivity was pre-set to 200 ng/ml, which is reflected in the results shown in Table 1. Greater sensitivity can be achieved with this method (HI) by using more dilute antiserum. The manufacturer and others[4] report that a sensitivity of 30 ng/ml may be achieved.

APPROPRIATE CUTOFF
CONCENTRATION

The great sensitivity of the immunoassays for

*The Department of Biochemistry, Case Western Reserve University, generously allowed the use of their scintillation counting equipment.
†Under the direction of Mr. Loren Price and Dr. James Larsen.

TABLE 1

Assay Responses

The average value and standard deviation of the response of each method to ten samples of morphine at each of the concentrations are listed. All samples were prepared from a single pool of methadone urine.

		Concentration (ng morphine/ml)					
Method	Response measured	0	100	200	400	600	1000
RIA*	Average counts ^{3}H/2 min/0.5 ml	7,610 ±180	8,780 ±220	9790 ±380	11,370 ±270	12,410 ±350	13,400 ±480
FRAT	Average peak height (mm)	27 ±2	41 ±3	54 ±2	69 ±4	82 ±3	95 ±4
EMIT	Average decrease in absorbance (436 nm)	.018 ±.002	.020 ±.002	.023 ±.002	.033 ±.002	.041 ±.003	.058 ±.003
HI**	Number samples neg.	10	1	0	0	0	0
	Number samples ±	0	5	1	0	0	0
	Number samples pos.	0	4	9	10	10	10

*All samples were diluted 1/10 prior to analysis by RIA, since quantitative results cannot be obtained by this method at concentrations greater than 60 to 100 ng/ml.

**The antiserum was diluted to yield a sensitivity of 200 ng/ml for the HI test.

morphine, especially RIA and HI, which can detect levels of 10 to 30 ng/ml, raises the issue of whether values in this very low range are significant. An empirical approach to this problem is to assay by RIA a large number of drug-free urines in order to define the upper limits of the responses produced by negative samples. Catlin et al.[5] have reported that of 171 urines obtained from healthy drug-free individuals, 97% contained less than 25 ng morphine equivalents (ME)/ml. However, the majority of samples analyzed by our laboratory were not obtained from drug-free individuals, but from ex-addicts enrolled in drug rehabilitation programs (in which the use of methadone and a variety of sedatives and tranquilizers is commonplace) or from patients admitted to local hospitals. Therefore, in order to estimate an appropriate cutoff limit for urines of this type, 738 (undiluted) samples from patients in several such rehabilitation clinics were analyzed by RIA. It was assumed *a priori* that a large majority of these samples would not contain morphine, and that these would produce a distribution of values near zero which could be distinguished from the distribution of morphine-positive samples. The data presented in Figure 1 reveal a sharp distinction between the large number of samples (assumed to be morphine-free) between 0 and 100 ng/ml and all those at concentrations greater than 100 ng/ml. Thus we suggest an appropriate cutoff limit between positive and negative morphine results by RIA (and also HI) should be no less than 100 ng/ml and preferably somewhat higher. The manufacturer of RIA (Hoffmann-LaRoche) currently recommends a cutoff level of 100 ng/ml, which seems appropriate.

A similar graphical analysis of the EMIT responses to the same 738 samples analyzed by RIA (Figure 1A) is presented in Figure 1B. In this case, the appropriate cutoff limit appears to be a minimum decrease in absorbance of .060 to .070. This corresponds to an apparent morphine concentration of 600 to 800 ng/ml, which is in basic agreement with the limit recommended by the manufacturer (Syva Corporation). The cutoff limit for FRAT, based on a similar study by the Syva Corporation, is 500 ng/ml. These results are summarized in Table 2. The use of these relatively high cutoff values assumes the risk that authentic positive samples at concentrations lower than these limits will not be detected, but it has the merit that large numbers of false positive results will be excluded. In addition, several non-immunological techniques (TLC, fluorometry, and

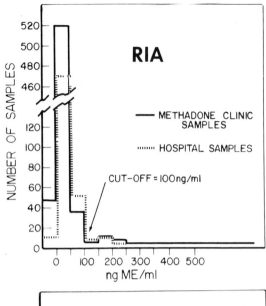

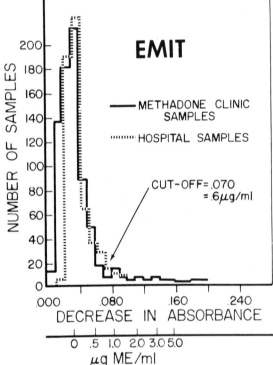

FIGURE 1. Normal background. The frequency distribution of the responses of RIA and EMIT to a number of urine samples which were obtained from populations in which a majority of the individuals were not receiving heroin or morphine. Most of the samples produce responses which form a distribution around the average response of negative controls. The width of the distribution is taken to reflect the normal range of responses produced by negative samples. The "cutoff" response or concentration is selected such that a large majority (90 to 95%) of these samples produce responses which are below the "cutoff."

GLC) have similar sensitivity limits (100 to 600 ng/ml), and so may be used to confirm the presence of morphine in those samples that do fall above the recommended cutoff limits.

Accuracy and Precision

The precision of each of the quantitative methods is reflected in the magnitude of the standard deviations listed in Table 1. As may be seen, precision is relatively high for all methods (± 3 to 10%) throughout the concentration range studied.

Because the standard curves for all immunoassays are nonlinear, the accuracy with which results such as those in Table 1 can be translated into the corresponding concentration values is a function principally of two factors: (a) how accurately the standard curve is known and (b) on what portion of the standard curve the value lies. For the conversion of the data reported in Table 1, standard curves were prepared by assaying known aliquots of the same six solutions of morphine that were assayed as unknowns. Consequently, good accuracy was achieved as shown in Table 3. Under normal circumstances, the manufacturers recommend standard curves of only three or four concentrations. These approximate the true standard curves only moderately well, and accuracy under these conditions will be lower than that indicated in Table 3, but nonetheless may still be acceptable.

Specificity

One of the most important advantages of the immunoassays is that they measure drugs in urine directly, without prior extraction, purification, or concentration of drug from the urine. This is based on the inherent sensitivity and specificity of these methods. However, this specificity is not absolute and other drugs or molecules of similar structure may cross-react. The degree to which other substances will cross-react is a function of the specificity of the antisera used which, in turn, is a function of the technique used to produce the antisera. Of particular importance is the structure of the drug-protein antigen used to induce antibody synthesis. While an extensive evaluation of the specificity of the antisera supplied with each of the four immunoassays for morphine was beyond the scope of this project, other authors have reported their findings on this question, and their data are summarized in Table 4. As may be

TABLE 2
Sensitivity

A listing of the maximum sensitivity of each method and the recommended lower limit (cutoff) which should be applied to define positive and negative samples.

Method	Maximum sensitivity	Appropriate cutoff conc.
RIA	10 ng/ml	100 ng/ml
FRAT	100 ng/ml	500 ng/ml
EMIT	400 ng/ml	600 ng/ml
HI	30 ng/ml	100–200 ng/ml

TABLE 3
Assay Precision

The average value and standard deviation of the concentration values obtained by assaying 10 samples of urine containing morphine sulfate at each of the six concentrations indicated.

Method	Concentration (ng/ml)					
	0	100	200	400	600	1,000
RIA	0 ±30	120 ±30	210 ±50	400 ±70	690 ±140	1,200 ±300
FRAT	0 ±20	120 ±30	220 ±30	410 ±30	620 ±60	1,080 ±200
EMIT	0 ±100	80 ±80	180 ±50	420 ±60	590 ±70	980 ±70

TABLE 4
Interferences

Some of the compounds tested for cross-reactivity in the four morphine immunoassay systems. The relative reactivity of a compound is the response of that compound divided by the response of an equal concentration of morphine. These data were obtained from those references indicated.

Substance	Relative reactivity			
	RIA[6]	FRAT[7]	EMIT[9]	HI[4]
Morphine	1.00	1.00	1.00	+
Codeine	1.1	5.00	1.5	+
Morphine glucuronide	0.8	0.99[8]	0.90	+
Methadone	.001	.001	.001	−
Meperidine	.002	.014	.030	+
Dextromethorphan	.001	.003	.007	±
Propoxyphene	0	.001	.007	±
Dihydrocodinone	N.A.*	0.3–3.0[8]	N.A.	N.A.
Dihydromorphinone	N.A.	N.A.	N.A.	+
Nalorphine	.001	.059	.180	N.A.
Chlorpromazine	.001	.002	.006	−
Poppy seeds	+	N.A.	+	+

*N.A. = data not available.

seen, the cross-reactivity of most drugs is semi-quantitatively similar in each of the assays.

Strong Cross-reactors

Of the variety of compounds which react strongly with morphine antiserum of this type, codeine and morphine glucuronide are most significant. This reaction with morphine glucuronide is a distinct advantage since most of the total morphine in urine exists as the glucuronide. However, the strong cross-reaction with codeine is a marked disadvantage because it is a legitimate drug that is commonly used, and hence it is the most probable source of false positive tests for morphine by immunoassay.

A number of synthetic morphine analogues such as nalorphine, ethyl morphine, dihydromorphinone, and dihydrocodeinone also cross-react well. However, the frequency of the therapeutic use or the abuse of these drugs is relatively low so that instances of false positives due to these drugs should be infrequent. Of importance is the low but significant cross-reactivity due to some unknown substance(s) found in poppyseeds. In a single experiment in our laboratory, urine from a drug-free individual who ate one piece of poppyseed strudel was found to exceed the cutoff response when assayed by RIA and EMIT, and was positive by HI.

Poor Cross-reactors

Other common narcotics such as methadone and meperidine (Demerol) as well as other important drugs such as dextromethorphan and chlorpromazine cross-react quite poorly so that false positive results from these substances, if any, would occur only at the very high concentrations resulting from acute exposures.

In view of the number of compounds which do give positive reactions, even if only a few of them are likely to be encountered, *it is mandatory that all positive results by any immunoassay be confirmed by one or more non-immunological techniques of equivalent sensitivity.*

RELIABILITY

One criterion of the reliability of an assay is its agreement with other comparable assays. In order to estimate the reliability of the immunoassays under clinical conditions, 165 samples were assayed in parallel by each of the four techniques. Taking into consideration the differences in

TABLE 5

Assay Agreement

The frequency with which one method was found to give a result judged to be inconsistent with the results of the other three methods (165 samples were assayed by each technique).

Method	% Internal inconsistency
RIA	1.8%
FRAT	1.2%
EMIT	1.8%
HI	3.6%

appropriate cutoff levels (Table 2), a tabulation was made of instances in which one method gave a result which was judged to be inconsistent with the result of the other three methods. The results are summarized in Table 5. As indicated, the four immunoassays show good internal agreement. Reassay of samples which were in internal disagreement generally resolved the discrepancy, indicating the most common source of these discrepancies was operator error, rather than sample or assay idiosyncrasy.

TIME

The time required to perform an assay is a function of the extent to which semi-fully automated equipment is incorporated into the procedure. The values reported in Table 6 were derived by using only the standard equipment associated with each assay, and following the manufacturer's prescribed procedures.

COST

The usual cost of instruments and other hardware and of reagents and disposable items is listed in Table 7. The cost of reagents will frequently depend upon the quantity of material purchased, since most manufacturers offer a reduced unit price to large volume users.

OTHER DRUGS

Reagents for the detection of drugs other than morphine, including amphetamine, methadone, barbiturates, and benzoylecgonine, are currently available for the EMIT and FRAT systems. The performance of the EMIT system in the detection

TABLE 6

Assay Time

A summary of the time factors with respect to the analysis of samples by each of the immunoassays, using the standard equipment associated with each assay, and following the manufacturers' directions.

		Time (min)	
Method	1 Assay	100 Assays	Samples/day/operator
RIA	60–90	200–250	200–300
FRAT	1	100–120	400–500
EMIT	1	150–200	200–300
HI	120–180	200–250	200–300

TABLE 7

Assay Costs

Approximate cost ranges for instruments and reagents and other disposable items for each of the immunoassays.

Method	Cost of instruments and hardware	Cost per test of reagents and disposables
RIA	$ 7,000–15,000	$.50–1.00*
FRAT	$26,000	$.50–1.00
EMIT	$ 6,500	$.50–.90
HI	$ 0	$.30–.40

*When ^{125}I-labeled material is used, the cost of reagents is lower since no scintillation fluid or vial is used.

of these drugs was evaluated by comparing the results of EMIT analyses with the results of GLC or TLC analyses of the same urine samples. The results are summarized in the following set of tables.

Methadone

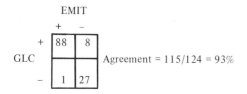

EMIT

GLC

Agreement = 115/124 = 93%

Of the eight samples identified as positive by GLC and negative by EMIT, three were at low concentration (400 to 600 ng/ml), at or near the sensitivity limit of EMIT for methadone (500 ng/ml). The remaining five samples appear to be authentic false negatives. One advantage of GLC

(or TLC) for the identification of methadone is that it also identifies the major metabolite of methadone (2-ethylidene-1,5-dimethyl-3,3-diphenylpyrrolidine) while the EMIT assay does not. In this group of 124 samples, five were identified by GLC as methadone positive on the basis of the presence of the metabolite, even though the methadone concentration was very low or absent. Since the EMIT system does not detect this metabolite of methadone, for the purposes of this comparison these 5 cases were listed among the 27 methadone negatives by GLC.

Amphetamine

EMIT

GLC

Agreement = 193/211 = 89%

The 11 samples identified as positive by GLC and negative by EMIT were at or below the detection limit of the EMIT system for amphetamine (3,000 ng/ml). The 13 samples identified as positive by EMIT and negative by GLC are probably due to cross-reacting amines such as phenylpropanolamine or other common ingredients of cold pills. A "back-up reagent," intended to reduce the incidence of such cross-reaction, did not seem to be effective.

Barbiturates

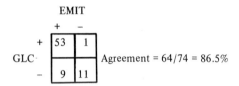

As with the amphetamine reagent, there are a significant number of samples identified as positive by EMIT but negative by GLC. Again, this may be due to cross-reacting nonbarbiturates, or it may be due to reaction of metabolites of the barbiturates which are not extracted into toluene and/or are not identified by GLC.

Benzoylecgonine and/or Cocaine

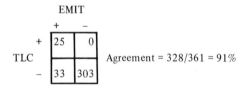

Cocaine is metabolized in man to benzoylecgonine and ecgonine. The use of cocaine by an individual may be detected by TLC by the presence in the urine of any or all of these three compounds, while the EMIT reagent is relatively specific for benzoylecgonine (sensitivity limit around 1,000 ng/ml). Thus the possibility exists that the EMIT system would fail to detect samples containing cocaine (or ecgonine) which were low in benzoylecgonine, and these samples might be detected by TLC. The data above indicate that the frequency of such samples is low since no sample that was identified as cocaine positive by TLC was found to be negative by EMIT. That is, if there is sufficient cocaine to be detected by TLC there will also be sufficient benzoylecgonine to be detected

by EMIT. The 33 samples identified as positive by EMIT but negative by TLC may well represent samples below the detection level of TLC for cocaine/benzoylecgonine. Thus, the EMIT system appears to be the most sensitive (and reliable) method for the detection of cocaine abuse, even though presently available techniques may not be able to confirm low positive samples.

SUMMARY OF EMIT/GLC/TLC COMPARISON

The four preceding tables indicate that there is generally good agreement (86 to 93%) between EMIT and GLC or TLC with respect to the analysis of amphetamine, barbiturates, methadone, and benzoylecgonine (cocaine). The principal discrepancies are of two types: (1) superior sensitivity of one method over the other and (2) probable cross-reacting material which leads to false positives by the EMIT system, again underscoring the principle that all immunological positive results must be confirmed by nonimmunological techniques.

DISCUSSION

The immunotechniques are powerful and useful new additions to the methods currently available to the analytical toxicologist. As a group, their principal advantage is their ability to detect drugs of abuse in urine directly without prior extraction and concentration of the drugs from the urine.

Their major limitation, due to the cross-reactivity of a large number of compounds, is that positive results are ambiguous, and must be confirmed by one or more nonimmunological techniques. On the other hand, all negative results are highly reliable, down to the limits of sensitivity for each method. Therefore, all negative samples may be excluded from further consideration, and only positive samples need be tested further. Another important limitation of immunoassays is that they can test for only one drug (or one class of drugs) at a time, as opposed to chromatographic methods such as TLC and GLC which can test for a large number of drugs simultaneously. When it is necessary to assay for several drugs in each sample, the cost and time per sample of the immunoassays will increase correspondingly. Theoretically, by combining the reagents for the detection of several different drugs into one "polyvalent" immuno-

TABLE 8
Relative Cost/Time Factors

	Number of drugs tested simultaneously			
Percent positive* samples	2	3	4	5
1	1.02	1.03	1.04	1.05
5	1.10	1.15	1.20	1.25
10	1.20	1.30	1.40	1.50
20	1.40	1.60	1.80	2.00

*A positive result would indicate the presence of any one or more of the drugs included in the combined assay.

assay, the increase in cost and time can be limited (especially in those situations where the incidence of positive samples is low), although the net cost and time per sample will still be higher than for the analysis for a single drug. Table 8 indicates the relationship between the relative increase in the cost/time factor, the number of drugs combined in one test, and the frequency of positive samples. The relative increase in cost would depend upon the price of the reagents for the combined assay system. Whether polyvalent immunoassays are practical and feasible is yet to be determined.

Thus, the proper role of immunoassays appears to be as a screening technique for the presence of a single drug, or possibly two or three other specific drugs. Under these conditions the time and cost per sample may still be competitive with TLC or GLC. When it is necessary to identify a larger number of drugs, immunoassays generally will not be useful as screening techniques, although they may still be valuable as confirmatory methods. An important consideration with respect to this point is that the most recent federal guidelines[10] for minimal surveillance of individuals in methadone maintenance programs involves testing for drugs other than morphine only once per month. Should this approach be adopted, the immunoassays are well suited as a primary screening technique for morphine.

Although the immunoassays as a group are similar in many respects, each of the four commercially available techniques offers unique features. In summary, a brief review of these features as well as some subjective comments concerning each assay is presented below.

RIA

This method is the most sensitive technique available for the detection of morphine. In fact, the method is so sensitive that it is frequently necessary to dilute positive samples by factors of 1/5 to 1/500 in order to obtain quantitative results. Although the assay procedure involves many operations, it is simple to perform. Relatively slow for small numbers of samples, the average time per sample is low (2 to 3 min) when large numbers (100 to 300) are analyzed. Reagent costs ($0.50 to $1.00/test) are competitive with other immunoassays. Instrument costs (for a gamma or liquid scintillation count) are high ($7,000 to $15,000) but the instrument may be of general usefulness, since radioimmunoassays are available for a variety of compounds[11] and radioactively labeled drugs are available for many research applications. Use of radioactive isotopes creates some problems with respect to licensing, handling, and disposing of the radioactive material, but these are not serious drawbacks. The use of these reagents involves practically no radiation hazard from the amounts of radioactivity involved. The shelf-life of the ^{125}I-labeled morphine is limited (half-life 56 days), but the ^{3}H-labeled reagent is relatively stable. Use of the ^{125}I reagent is faster, easier and less expensive than the ^{3}H-labeled material, since no scintillation fluid or vial is required.

EMIT

The principal advantage of this method is its capacity for rapid analyses (approximately one minute per sample), which may be of particular value in certain clinical and legal situations. Since reagents are currently available for morphine, methadone, amphetamine, barbiturates, and benzoylecgonine, this system is also the most versatile at this time. The cost of reagents ($0.50 to $0.90 per test) is comparable to the RIA, but instrument costs are considerably lower (around $7,000). While the sensitivity of EMIT for morphine (500 to 600 ng/ml) is not as high as the sensitivity of RIA or HI, this level may be acceptable for most applications. Since the EMIT assay depends on the activity of an enzyme (lysozyme) whose pH optimum is 6 to 7, urine samples that are especially alkaline (as a result of bacterial action during prolonged storage, 5 to 15 days at room temperature) may exceed the buffering capacity of the system and result in reduced sensitivity. Under these circumstances it is necessary to buffer the urines to pH 6 to 7 before assay. Endogenous lysozyme in urine is a possible source of false positives, but these may be eliminated by the use of proper controls. Of all the immunoassays, EMIT is the most easily automated. When available, this promises to result in even faster analyses at lower cost per test.

FRAT

The FRAT system is similar to EMIT in many respects, but the very high instrument cost ($26,000), plus the limited usefulness of an ESR spectrometer to most toxicology laboratories, renders this technique useful only to laboratories performing many analyses per day.

HI

Very inexpensive (instrument cost $0, reagent cost $0.30/test) and quite sensitive (30 ng/ml), this procedure is very promising. A major drawback is that the results must be judged subjectively, and interpretation may vary from individual to individual. In addition, manual delivery of samples and reagents into the reaction well is tedious and error prone, but automation of these operations may relieve this problem. Quite slow (2 to 3 hr) for small numbers of samples, it is comparable to other immunoassays for larger numbers of samples (200 to 300/day/operator).

Currently, there is considerable variability in the properties of antisera and sensitized red blood cells, and careful monitoring of all reagents is required in order to insure adequate performance. These problems are encountered most frequently when prediluted antiserum is used, probably as a result of loss of antibody activity. By using a concentrated stock solution of antibody and titrating it each day with the red blood cells that will be used that day, the method is quite reliable. Daily titration is time consuming and involves some effort, but its advantages (increased reliability, plus the capacity to select the sensitivity desired) definitely warrant this step. Improvements in the production of morphine-labeled red blood cells have been reported by the developer. This may eliminate the variability in this reagent and increase the overall reproducibility of the technique.

ACKNOWLEDGMENTS

This work was supported in part by funds provided by Grant 9863-11 from the National Institute of General Medical Sciences. The support of Roche Diagnostics (RIA), SYVA Company (EMIT and FRAT) and Materials and Technology Systems, Inc. (HI), as well as the cooperation of United Medical Laboratories (for FRAT analyses), is gratefully acknowledged.

REFERENCES

1. **Kananen, G., Osiewicz, R., and Sunshine, I.,** Barbiturate analysis, a current assessment, *J. Chromatogr. Sci.,* 10, 283, 1972.
2. **Aggarwal, V., Bath, R., and Sunshine, I.,** in press, *Clin. Chem.,* Feb., 1974.
3. **Davidow, B., Li Petri, N., and Quame, B.,** A thin-layer chromatographic screening procedure for detecting drug abuse, *Am. J. Clin. Pathol.,* 50, 714, 1968.
4. **Adler, F. L., Liu, C. T., and Catlin, D.,** Methodology and application of a hemagglutination test for the detection of morphine, *Clin. Immunol. Immunopathol.,* 1, 53, 1972.
5. **Catlin, D., Cleeland, R., and Grunberg, E.,** A sensitive rapid radioimmunoassay for morphine and immunologically related substances in urine and serum, *Clin. Chem.,* 19, 216, 1973.
6. Data supplied by Diagnostic Research, Hoffmann-La Roche Inc., Nutley, N.J.
7. Syva Co., *FRAT Opiate Assay,* Palo Alto, Calif., October, 1972.
8. **Dubowski, K.,** Free radical assay techniques for drugs, *Ann. Clin. Lab. Sci.,* 1, 199, 1971.
9. Syva Co., *EMIT Enzyme Immunoassay System,* Palo Alto, Calif., 27, June, 1972.
10. Title 21, Food and drugs, in the Federal Register, Vol. 37, No. 242, Chap. I, part 130, Dec. 15, 1972.
11. **Skelly, D. S., Brown, L. P., and Besch, P. K.,** Radioimmunoassay, *Clin. Chem.,* 19, 146, 1973.

SUMMARY OF RECENT STUDIES OF THE VALIDITY OF METHODS OF DETECTION OF DRUGS OF ABUSE IN BIOLOGICAL FLUIDS

C. W. Gorodetzky

TABLE OF CONTENTS

INTRODUCTION

A major interest in our laboratory has been the study of the validity of methods of detection of drugs of abuse in biological fluids. Here, validity means the ability of a method to detect a drug or its metabolites in biological fluids following drug administration to humans. Validity pertains to answering the important clinical question: How long after a given dose of a drug by a given route of administration can a specified method continue to detect the drug or its metabolites in biological fluids (e.g. urine)? Although knowledge of a method's validity is essential to its intelligent use and interpretation, there has been little systematic study of this parameter. Whereas most other attempts to estimate the time course of detection of drugs of abuse by various methodologies have involved evaluation of clinical samples, where the nature, dose, route, and time of drug administration were known only by history, our approach has been an experimental one, in which these parameters are known with certainty. We have recently completed two studies on the validity of several methods to detect morphine in urine following single intravenous doses of heroin and morphine.

EXPERIMENTAL DESIGN

The subjects for all of our studies were healthy, adult, male federal prisoner volunteers from whom informed consent was obtained. All are former narcotic addicts who were incarcerated at the National Institute of Mental Health Addiction Research Center at the time of the study. All had not received chronic drug administration for at least 3 months and had been off all drugs for at least 3 weeks prior to the study. During the study they were housed on the research ward under close supervision.

In the first study,[1,2] two single intravenous doses of heroin, 2.5 and 5.0 mg/70 kg, were administered at weekly intervals in random order to 10 subjects. Since the average "street dose" of heroin appears to be highly variable and could not be determined with any accuracy, the doses chosen for the study were based on pharmacologic criteria. These doses have been found to be minimally to moderately euphorogenic in non-tolerant man.[3] They are also within the range of reported illicit heroin purchases on the street.[4] In the second study,[5] two single intravenous doses of morphine, 6 and 12 mg/70 kg (equieuphorogenic to the doses of heroin used in the first study)[3] were administered as described above to a second group of 10 subjects.

Prior to drug administration, two 24-hr urine collections were made to serve as negative controls. Following each drug administration, urine samples were collected for 1 week; all urines were collected ad lib, and in addition, each subject was asked to urinate every 8th hr. No special food or water restrictions were maintained in an attempt to provide a normal living environment. At the end of the 1-week collection period, the urine samples from each subject were combined into approximately 4- to 8-hr samples to give sufficient volume in each so that the desired chemical tests could be performed.

CHEMICAL METHODS

All samples plus aliquots of the pre-drug control urines (and in some cases aliquots of pooled normal urine) were randomized, coded, and analyzed under blind conditions by each of seven different methods: four separate extraction procedures (organic solvent and ion exchange resin impregnated paper extraction both with and without prior acid hydrolysis) followed by thin-layer chromatography (TLC) using iodoplatinate spray for identification; the Technicon® Autoanalyzer; the free radical assay technique (FRAT®) and the radioimmunoassay (RIA). The latter three analyses were performed in collaboration with Drs. Angel, Beach, and Catlin at the Walter Reed Army Institute of Research. The TLC procedures were modifications of the organic solvent procedure described by Mulé and the ion exchange resin paper extraction of Dole.[6] These methods have a sensitivity of 0.1 to 0.25 μg morphine per ml of urine. The Technicon Autoanalyzer analyses[7] were performed on a prototype instrument supplied to the Walter Reed Army Institute of Research. A

sample was considered positive if its reading exceeded that of an 0.2 μg/ml urinary morphine standard. In the FRAT analyses,[8] the total opiate antisera was used. Data were analyzed using two cutoffs for positives: (1) greater than the 0.5 μg/ml aqueous morphine standard (as recommended by the manufacturer), and (2) greater than the upper $P = .05$, 95% tolerance limits[9] of the known negative urines run under blind conditions on the same day. The latter analysis was undertaken since the experimental samples were old at the time of analysis and not preadjusted for pH or ionic strength (factors which were found subsequent to analysis to be a possible source of false-positives). Both analyses gave qualitatively similar results, but the latter analysis gave considerably fewer false-positives. The radioimmunoassay was based on the work of Spector and Parker[10] and performed according to the detailed procedure described by Catlin.[11] A sample was considered positive if its reading exceeded that of a 50-ng/ml urinary morphine standard.

Results were tabulated as the percent of urine samples positive in each 8-hr period following drug administration. Percent false-positives were based on the analysis of the predrug control and pooled normal urine samples.

RESULTS

In the heroin study, using both TLC procedures without hydrolysis there was a high proportion of positives (greater than 70%) for only the first 8 hr following administration of both doses. Using these procedures with prior acid hydrolysis, there was a high proportion of positives for 8 hr following the low dose and 8 to 16 hr following the high dose. The Technicon Autoanalyzer results showed a high proportion of positives for only the first 8 hr following only the high dose of heroin. The FRAT results were very similar to those using ion exchange resin-impregnated paper extraction and TLC with hydrolysis, showing a high proportion of positives for 8 hr following the low heroin dose and 16 hr following the high dose. The radioimmunoassay gave 90 to 100% positives for 32 hr following the low dose and 40 hr following the high dose, falling to about 80% positive at 48 hr following the high dose.

In the morphine experiment, TLC procedures without hydrolysis gave a high proportion of positives for 8 hr following the low morphine dose and 8 to 16 hr following the high dose. With prior acid hydrolysis, the TLC procedures showed a high proportion of positives for 32 hr following the low dose and 32 to 48 hr following the high dose. The Technicon Autoanalyzer results showed a high proportion of positives for only the first 8 hr following both morphine doses. The FRAT analysis gave a high proportion of positives for 32 hr following the low dose and 48 hr following the high dose. Using radioimmunoassay, there were 100% positives for 40 hr following the low dose, falling to 60 to 85% from the 48th hr through the 72nd hr; following the high morphine dose there were 90 to 100% positives for 72 hr, and about 50% positives during the 4th day. False-positives were: 0% for the radioimmunoassay, organic solvent extraction without hydrolysis, and both ion exchange resin impregnated paper extractions; 1% for FRAT; 2.5% for organic solvent extraction with hydrolysis; and, 3% for the Technicon Autoanalyzer.

SUMMARY

Following minimally to moderately euphorogenic doses of heroin, our study showed a high probability of detection of morphine in the urine for 8 hr using TLC procedures without hydrolysis and the Technicon Autoanalyzer, for 8 to 16 hr using TLC procedures with hydrolysis and FRAT, and for 32 to 48 hr using radioimmunoassay. Following equieuphorogenic doses of morphine, there was a high probability of detection of morphine in the urine for 8 to 16 hr using TLC procedures without hydrolysis and the Technicon Autoanalyzer, 32 to 48 hr using TLC procedures with hydrolysis and the FRAT, and 72 hr using the radioimmunoassay. We anticipate continuation of validity studies in our laboratory to provide data on other drugs of abuse, new methodologies, and biological fluids other than urine (e.g. saliva and plasma).

REFERENCES

1. Gorodetzky, C. W., Time course of morphine (M) detection in human urine after IV heroin (H), *Fed. Proc. Abstr.*, 31, 528, 1972.
2. Gorodetzky, C. W., Angel, C. R., Beach, D. J., Catlin, D. H., and Yeh, S., Validity of screening methods for drugs of abuse in biological fluids. I. Heroin in urine, *Clin. Pharmacol. Ther.*, in press.
3. Martin, W. R. and Fraser, H. F., A comparative study of physiological and subjective effects of heroin and morphine administered intravenously in postaddicts, *J. Pharmacol. Exp. Ther.*, 133, 388, 1961.
4. Moore, J. M. and Bena, F. E., Rapid gas chromatographic assay for heroin in illicit preparations. *Anal. Chem.*, 44, 385, 1972.
5. Gorodetzky, C. W., Time course of morphine (M) detection in human urine after IV morphine, *Fed. Proc. Abstr.*, 32, 764, 1973.
6. Gorodetzky, C. W., Efficiency and sensitivity of two common screening methods for detecting morphine in urine, *Clin. Chem.*, 19, 753, 1973.
7. Sansur, M., Buccafuri, A., and Morgenstern, S., Automated fluorometric method for the determination of morphine in urine, *J. Assoc. Off. Anal. Chem.*, 55, 880, 1972.
8. Leute, R., Ullman, E., and Goldstein, A., Spin immunoassay of opiate narcotics in urine and saliva, *J.A.M.A.*, 221, 1231, 1972.
9. Goldstein, A., *Biostatistics: An introductory text,* Macmillan Co. New York, 1964, 49.
10. Spector, S. and Parker, C. W., Morphine radioimmunoassay, *Science,* 168, 1347, 1970.
11. Catlin, D., Cleeland, R., and Grunberg, E., A sensitive, rapid radioimmunoassay for morphine and immunologically related substances in urine and serum, *Clin. Chem.*, 19, 216, 1973.

DISCUSSION

The authors (Drs. Catlin, Mulé, Sunshine, and Gorodetzky) have described the effective use of each immunoassay technique as applied to the analysis of biological material for drugs subject to abuse. These studies emphasized certain concepts, some of which require further probing. Among these are validity, sensitivity, cross-reactivity (specificity), false positives, and false negatives. The validity of an assay is dependent upon the dose, the route of administration, biological material analyzed, and of course the sensitivity of the technique. Obviously the greater the sensitivity the more valid an assay will be in relation to duration of detection (i.e., hours, days, or weeks) after drug administration. Sensitivity of an assay may be defined in terms of total concentration (nanogram, microgram, etc.) or concentration per volume (microgram/ml), or the amount detected in a period of time (50 to 99%) with statistical verification. How sensitive a technique should be is dependent upon the needs of the user. The assay should be as sensitive as physically possible consistent with cost and specificity factors. Currently all immunoassays lack absolute specificity so that many chemically related compounds cross-react within a given assay. All comparisons of cross-reactive compounds should be on an equivalent basis, for example, a test concentration of a drug or metabolite which reacts in a certain immunoassay equivalent to 1 μg of morphine. The data may also be calculated as a ratio relative to the standard morphine. In this way all laboratories may readily compare the cross-reactivity (specificity) of the immunoassay for the chemical tested. Certainly, it would appear at first glance that false-positive or negative samples would be self-explanatory. This is not so. All false determinations are relative, and are related to known conditions or to a standard analytical technique, which in turn has certain limitations. For example, in an analysis where the investigator has full control over drug administration and collection of the biological material or adds drugs to these materials or is *certain* the material contains no drugs, then a false-positive determination would be indicative of a faulty technique (or one exceedingly sensitive) or technical error. A false-negative under these conditions would indicate limitations in sensitivity of the method or again technical error. Where the analysis is performed on a totally unknown sample, then a false determination must be in reference to a standard analytical technique. In this case, the reference method should, if at all possible, be the most sensitive and specific available. Gas chromatography coupled with mass spectrometry (GCMS) provides the required sensitivity and specificity to confirm the presence of drugs in biological material (see article by Dr. Hawk). Certain problems concerning purification of the sample may exist, but GCMS essentially meets the requirements to support and/or confirm the data received from all immunoassays. Certainly, other analytical techniques, i.e., gas, liquid, or thin layer chromatography, and fluorometry, may be used to confirm the results of immunoassays, provided the comparative sensitivity limitations between the analytical techniques and the immunoassays are well understood. It must be further emphasized that one immunoassay cannot be used to confirm the results from other immunoassays, due to the lack of specificity (cross-reactivity) peculiar to all immunoassays. Although confirmation of a positive result is essential, a negative determination may be readily accepted. In fact, the immunoassays appear to be excellent exclusion tests for drugs subject to abuse.

The cost of the analysis is important and is related to use of the data. In the case of legal or forensic implications cost should not be a major factor and all immunoassay results should be confirmed by one or more analytical techniques other than immunological. For routine screening of vast numbers of samples, cost must be kept to a minimum and additional confirmatory tests are not required provided the data are utilized only as a means of further and specific counseling of the individual. In punitive programs where a significant reduction in freedom of the individual is at stake or loss of employment is involved, then certainly additional confirmatory tests are mandatory, even though an increased cost is incurred.

An important concern of any analytical laboratory is quality control. Good laboratories exercise internal controls on all analyses whether they be for routine or for research purposes. However, some laboratories are not so motivated. In order to maintain quality control, proficiency testing was initiated at the federal level through the Center for Disease Control (CDC) and through various state controlled programs. A laboratory analyzing urines for drugs subject to abuse must meet certain minimal requirements in this area of toxicological analysis, regardless of the methods employed.

The future of immunochemistry as applied to clinical and analytical chemistry certainly appears bright. It seems the direction and emphasis of future research should be on the development of specific antibodies (antisera) for a given immunogen, so that cross-reactivity to a drug and/or metabolite is minimized. The idea of developing a multiple drug reagent whereby an immunoassay may be conducted for several drugs at the same time is also highly desirable. With a multiple reagent, a negative result would eliminate the need for further analysis, thus saving considerable time and money. A positive result would require additional tests for each drug.

Although the need for new immunoassay systems does not appear to be desirable at present, research efforts to develop more sensitive or specific systems should not be discouraged. New immunoassays for different drugs must be constantly considered in view of the changing social problem. This means development of only those assays for drugs which appear to *consistently* interrupt our social and legal system and for the newer chemotherapeutic agents (i.e., narcotic antagonists) should be given priority. To attempt to develop a new immunoassay for each and every drug in vogue would be both expensive and unjustified.

Automation of currently available systems for immunoassay should be avidly pursued. This is especially important to those laboratories required to analyze large numbers of samples on a daily basis. Furthermore, an increase in the use of urinalysis for drugs subject to abuse in agonist and antagonist maintenance treatment programs, employment screening, athletic contests, the military, and for medico-legal purposes requires that rapid and accurate automated technology be available.

Finally, it must be stated that the application of immunochemistry to the analysis of drugs subject to abuse has been the single most important event in this field of analysis in the past decade.

INDEX

Homogeneous immunoassays, 46
  electron spin resonance label-immunoassay technique (see also FRAT), 46

I

Immune assays, 3
Immunoassay, 91, 93
  comparative performance studies, 93
    clinical studies, 94
    guidelines for application of, 94–95
    interpretation of results, 94
  enzyme-multiplied immunoassay technique (EMIT), 91
  free-radial assay technique (FRAT), 91
  hemagglutination inhibition, 91
  radioimmunoassay, 91
  techniques, III
    advantages, III
    amphetamine, III
    barbiturates, III
    cocaine, III
    high costs, III
    LSD, III
    mescaline, III
    methadone, III
    morphine, III
    rapid, III
    simple, III
Instrument requirements for RIA, 18
  gamma counters, 18
  liquid scintillation counters, 18
In vivo probes, 9
  active immunization with immunogen, 9
  passive introduction of antibody, 9

L

Labeled haptens, 28
  advantages, 29
  disadvantages, 30
  monovalent hapten, 28
  multivalent hapten, 28
Licensing requirements for radioactivity, 19
  ^{125}I, 19
  AEC, 19
  ^{3}H, 19

M

Manufacturers of GCMS, 83
  characteristics of GCMS systems, 83
Mass spectrometry, 73
  chemical ionization, 74–75
    of barbiturate, 77
    of cocaine, 75
    of methadone, 77
  electron bombardment, 73
  electronic impact fragmentation, 73–74, 77
    of cocaine, 76–77, 85
    of methadone, 77

ion separators, 73, 82
  magnetic sectors, 73
  quadrupole separators, 73, 82
  time-of-flight, 73
Methadone, 113
  EMIT vs GLC, 113
  maintenance treatment programs MMTP, III
  metabolite, 113
Microcrystallography, 85
Morphine, 2, 6, 108, 118
  validity studies, 118

N

New chemical techniques (see RIA, HI, EMIT, FRAT)
Nitrocellulose membrane technique, 31
  advantages, 33
  disadvantages, 34
  factors to be considered when setting up, 31
  principle, 31
  procedure, 31

P

Primary methods, III
  gas liquid chromatography, III
  thin-layer chromatography (TLC), III
  spectrofluorometry (SPE), 99–100

R

Radioimmunoassay (RIA), 82, 99–100, 118
  advantages, 25
  codeine, 31, 33
  cross-reactivity, 84
    diazepam, 84
    diphenylhydantonin, 84
    thyroxine, 84
  dihydrocodeine, 33
  dihydromorphine, 33
  disadvantages, 27
  factors governing antigen-antibody interactions, 24
  factors to be considered when setting up the technique, 25
  for morphine, 14
    cutoff level, 16
    evaluation, 16
    negative results, 16
    positive results, 16
    protocol, 14
    quantitative test, 16
  heroin, 33
  limitations of, 82
  mescaline, 30
  morphine, 24, 33
  principle of, 24
  role in forensic analysis, 82
  tetrahydrocannabinol, 28
Reliability (morphine), 112
  criterion of, 112
  internal agreement, 112